You agree to accept all risks of using the information presented inside this book.

You agree that by continuing to read this book, where appropriate and/or necessary, you shall consult a professional (including but not limited to your doctor, attorney, or financial advisor or such other advisor as needed) before using any of the suggested remedies, techniques, or information in this book.

Intermittent Fasting for Women

A complete guide for weight loss, support your hormones, for a healthy lifestyle and slow aging through the autophagy process without losing taste, easy for Beginners.

\-

The Quick Guide to Perfect Intermittent Fasting

[Melany Burns]

Legal & Disclaimer

Conclusion

Introduction

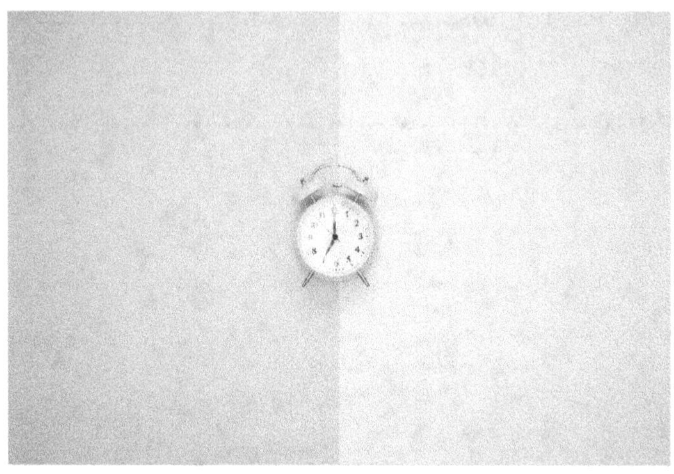

This book is going to change your life! I know you just started reading, but I'm serious! My book is designed to impact your life in the most positive way possible from a holistic standpoint.

You probably decided to buy this book because you want to become a better version of yourself! You made the best investment to invest in your health and wellness. I got good news for you, and that is your life will be transformed once you start taking action and implementing these strategies I discuss within this book.

Are you tired of being bombarded by countless infomercials that endorse new diet fads? I'm pretty sure you've heard it all from, ketogenic diet, paleo diet, vegan diet, and even the raw food diet. Now I'm not criticizing or taking jabs at any of these mentioned diets, and I do truly believe in most cases these diets do work effectively to a certain degree.

But you see there lies an inherent problem with all these so-called "diets." People tend to go on them and start seeing some results, but before you know it, they start gaining back those unwanted pounds simply because they couldn't uphold their regiment. To add insult to injury, a lot of these diets tend to be more costly and run an expensive bill that cannot be sustained on the average working person's budget.

Well, I'm here to tell you that intermittent fasting won't cost you any more than you are already spending. This diet, in particular, is designed to help you burn unwanted body fat fast and sculpt your way to your ideal physique in conjunction with exercise.

But, before we start discussing the basics, we need to get your mindset right! Something did not discuss a lot within the health and fitness industry, and that is having a good sense of self-awareness before you start any diet.

You see, the inherent problem I previously mentioned with all these diets is that people cannot uphold or continue on with certain diet regiments.

Why? Because people treat diets like prescription drugs! Once results are derived, and an outcome is finalized, people tend to go back to their old ways of living and relegate their newfound diet fad to the back burner.

You see, there is an inherent problem when you interface with a diet and consider it a short-term fix. True transformation takes place from the inside out, and when you become aware of changing the way you eat is not a matter of going on a short-term diet but a total lifestyle change!

That's right. You need to transform your lifestyle or modify it in order to achieve long term sustainable results! You need to incorporate intermittent fasting as apart of your daily living, and in order to do this, you need to shift your short term thinking to long term. This is not a prescription drug.

Obesity Epidemic – In Industrialized Societies

Studies have revealed that people found in the industrialized world (first world countries), in particular here in North America, have extremely high obesity rates. The Journal of the American Medical Association (JAMA) estimates that nearly 35.5% of women living in America are obese.

This rate has grown considerably over the past few years, especially ever since the advent of instant foods, fast foods, refined carbohydrates, and of course, sugary drinks, pastries, and other snacks.

Studies have revealed that people found in the industrialized world (first world countries), in particular here in North America, have extremely high obesity rates. The Journal of the American Medical Association (JAMA) estimates that nearly 35.5% of women living in America are obese.

This rate has grown considerably over the past few years, especially ever since the advent of instant foods, fast foods, refined carbohydrates, and of course, sugary drinks, pastries, and other snacks.

Now, I talked a lot about obesity rates among children and adults in most industrialized English-speaking countries tend to be abnormally high, and you know the reasons behind obesity stem from poor lifestyle choices, including lack of exercise and "Frankenstein foods."

But now let's do some compare and contrast, do you know which industrialized country has the lowest obesity rate and why? The answer is Japan! – That's right, a country that boasts as one of the world's leading technological powerhouses with advanced technology, relatively low crime rates, fast transportation, and let's not forget quality food!

So why do the Japanese have a much lower obesity rate in comparison to any other country of the industrialized parts of the world? The answer is simple, and that is their source of food! Japanese traditionally consume a lot of whole foods, while their counterparts the Americans eat foods that are heavily processed. It must be noted that American influence on Japanese cuisine is starting to infect Japanese people, but as a whole and generally speaking, the Japanese eat much cleaner.

Have you ever stopped to consider one of their most iconic foods, sushi? You can easily break down what traditional sushi is made up of; rice, raw fish or cooked fish, and seaweed. You can easily identify the components part by part, and this is what constitutes wholefoods!

Traditional sushi is made up of whole food ingredients, unlike our standard American "Frankenstein foods" that contain fillers, additives, preservatives, and artificial sweeteners. This simple but profound truth infers quite a lot. The fact is we need to start looking at our diets more closely and identify fake foods from authentic wholefoods.

The correlation between their low obesity rate and the consumption of whole foods is indisputable. Not only are whole foods packed with dense calories, but contain the essential vitamins, minerals, fibers, and other nutritional benefits that all human beings need to survive

Whole foods are plant-based foods that have little to minimal processing and have not undergone any acritical alterations.

Obesity is a serious thing. Obesity can be considered a jumping-off point to various chronic degenerative diseases; hence, why it is important to lose those unwanted pounds as quickly as possible. When you become overweight, you're at risk of a plethora of chronic disease states, such as cancer, diabetes, high blood pressure, stroke, gout, and even arthritis.

The dangers of obesity and being overweight cannot be understated. And I hope I was able to give you a quick summary in this introduction as to why you need to lose those unwanted pounds. Being overweight possesses certain health risks and complications that not only affect your self-esteem and body image but the outcome of your overall health too!

Chapter 1: Definition of Intermittent Fasting

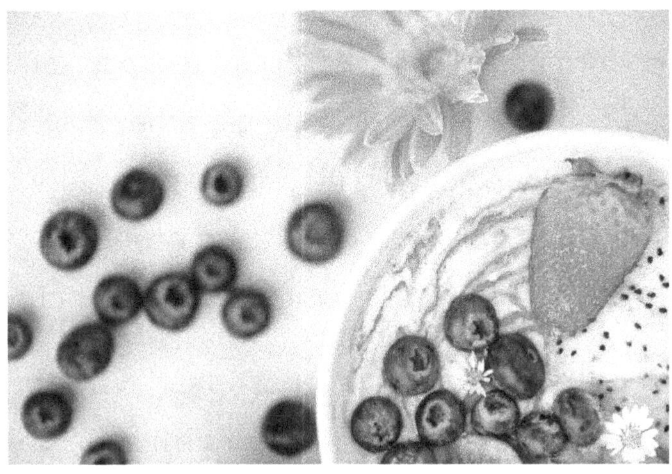

As stated earlier, in intermittent fasting, you have to go for long hours without eating any food. It can be done in several ways; skipping meals, Alternate-Day fasting, practicing the Eat-Stop-Eat method. Over the years, intermittent fasting has been helping women around the globe. Unfortunately, some women report that intermittent fasting has not been good for them as it has made them have binge consumptions, disruption of metabolic functioning, losing of the menstrual period, and having early menopause. Well, opting for intermittent fasting as a woman might appear as a little step to take in your life, but in the real sense, it comes along with huge impacts. Hormones that are responsible for regulating your ovulation are incredibly responsive to the energy consumption you have daily. Even the shortest term of fasting of about three days can alter a woman's hormones. Even the slightest acts of missing meals can change your emotions big time. It all depends on how quick your body is in responding to any change, and that is why you will find that some women can cope up with intermittent fasting while others cannot.

The notions bring up some questions: Why then does intermittent fasting affect female's hormone more than it does to the males? The best answer to this could be, Intermittent Fasting affects women more due to the effect brought about by the kisspeptin, which is a protein kind of molecule that is used by the neurons when communicating with each other. This molecule is sensitive to insulin and other hormones that are responsible for reacting to hunger or even satiety. Captivatingly, women's kisspeptin levels are higher as compared to those of any male mammal, and this translates to high sensitivities to any changes in energy balancing in the body.

There is a bigger intertwining between metabolism and the female reproductive system. A miss of the menstrual periods does not necessarily mean that you are pregnant; it can as well denote that your hormones have changed. Generally, females take in fewer proteins as compared to the males, a conditioned worsened by fasting. A less protein consumption means fewer intakes of amino acids required in the activation of estrogen, among other sex hormones. Low protein intakes can lead to reduced fertility in women. Estrogen hormone helps in the functioning of several parts in the body; brain, balancing of energy in the body, the formation of bones, healing, digestion, and even cognition. It means that women's bodies are more sensitive to energy changes and fertility.

Ways of Doing Intermittent Fasting

You can practice intermittent fasting in various ways. All that varies in these ways is the number of fasting days and the fat allowances. You should note that intermittent fasting entails having to abstain from taking any food for a specific set of hours before taking food regularly once more. These various ways will vary when it comes to every individual; each person's experience is unique in its way.

Fasting for Twelve Hours Each Day

In this diet, you have to follow simple rules of fasting for twelve hours every day. 10-16 hours fast helps your body in converting the fats into energy, and this, in turn, encourages losing bodyweight. Beginners of intermittent fasting are advised to start with this type of dieting. It is a simple way of fasting since, in most cases, you can do the fasting during the night or sleeping time and then take the same amount of fats every day. For instance, you can opt to take your dinner by 7 p.m. then sleep up to 7 a.m. so that you can have your breakfast. Including sleep in your fasting makes this method of doing recurrent starvation on yourself one of the simplest and easiest methods.

Fasting for Sixteen Hours

This is a way of intermittent fasting where you starve for sixteen hours to each time, then leave an eating space of eight hours. It is known as the Lean gains diet or the 16/8 way of fasting. For the women, you should fast for fourteen years, and have attempted the twelve hours fasting would be an added advantage to you. When doing this kind of dieting, you have to finish your meals by 8 p.m., skip breakfast the following day, and then take your lunch at around noon.

Fasting for Two Days Every Week

When following this way of intermittent fasting, you have to take health foods for five days and then decrease the fat consumption on the remaining two days. You can separate your fasting days in every week, but the fasting days should not follow each other. This kind of dieting reduces the levels of insulin in your body.

Weekly Twenty-Four-Hour Fasting

This is where you can fast for a whole day or two every week. You ensure that no food intake within twenty-four hours. You can opt for taking breakfasts or lunches each day within a week. Nonetheless, you can take drinks, tea, juice, water, and fat-free drinks when fasting. This way of fasting comes along with tiredness, headache, or even irritability since the body has not adjusted to the new system. But then again, if you have successfully practiced the twelve-hour or the sixteen-hour ways of fasting, it cannot be challenging to tolerate this kind of fasting.

Is intermittent fasting some new health fad that is taking the fitness industry by a storm, or is there more to it than meets the eye? What if I told you intermittent fasting isn't really something new!? But people have been practicing it since ancient times! That's right. Our ancestors didn't have supermarkets, fast food restaurant chains, or any other sources of quickly accessible food, and thus, as a result, were forced to interface with intermittent fasting on a daily basis.

Food was scantly available, and people didn't have the luxury of eating out on a whim or eating at their leisure. As a matter of fact, a point I wanted to highlight is people didn't eat out of boredom like we do today! Human beings are the only creatures on planet earth who eat out of boredom! Animals don't even do it!

Have you ever seen on wildlife documentaries prey such as buffalo or deer walking past content lions? Why don't the lions attack when they are content, and their bellies are filled? This is not a strange phenomenon, but a simple fact of life and that is animals only eat when they're hungry! Not out of boredom.

Human beings have acquired the habit of eating for either out of boredom, fun, stress, and other leisure times.

So you're probably wondering what is intermittent fasting, and how does it help you lose weight? Well, not only is it incredibly effective for helping you lose weight, but it is one of the best all-natural holistic healing solutions ever!

But before we get into the basics, we need to establish a few things. **1.** Fasting is not self-starvation, but volitionally choosing to use calorie restriction, eat less, and have your meals in fewer frequencies spread out at certain durations of the day. **2.** By intermittent fasting, you are restricting food intake for the first half of your day and then later introducing foods in the latter half. You essentially create windows of timeframes you fast under. **3.** Fasting has existed since ancient times and is completely healthy when done under the right supervision. You can fast for spiritual reasons, political reasons, or health-conscious reasons.

Fasting is a completely natural phenomenon that aligns itself with our normal physiological functions. In essence, fasting is a caloric restriction; in short, you are restricting the amount of calorie consumption you take in. But what does this do to the human body? IF (intermittent fasting) actually has quite a number of positive effects on our bodies, and this is backed by science. By intermittent fasting, we extend our life span, reverse the aging process, burns excess fat, enhances cardiovascular and brain health, reduce the risk of stroke, high blood pressure, oxidative stress, and improve insulin sensitivity.

You are probably wondering how on earth can fasting have so many benefits, and best of all, have no side effects like prescription drugs? Did I also mention that it is the most cost affordable solution for everybody on the planet! You can start completely FREE.

IF is when you don't eat for extended periods of time, unlike what we are taught to do by society's cultural norms, which is constantly eating. You create windows of "fasting," meaning you don't eat anywhere between 6-10-hour intervals, and the frequency of your eating is kept to 1-2 times a day or even eating every other day.

Now if you are starting out its going to be quite the task to readily jump into fasting for 12 hours straight, however, my advice is to build your way up, and note that the first week will probably be your hardest in regards to refraining from eating because your body is just starting to adapt and make the appropriate adjustments.

So, start off with six hours windows of not eating anything, and keep the frequency at two meals per day. Do this for the first week, and when you enter the second week, go for 8-hour windows and keep the frequency of eating the same. Once you've hit the 3rd week, I suggest either continuing your current regiment or step it up or notch to 10-hour intervals of abstinence and keep the frequency of 1 meal per day.

When you become comfortable, you can even take it to the next level, and that is eating every other day, meaning you don't eat at all for 24 hours that designated day. Thus, your only consuming food for four days out of a seven-day week. This equates to approximately 16 meals within a 30-day calendar month. Now, this is only for those of you who want to follow IF to this extreme; however, it's completely fine if you want to do two meals per day with 8-hour intervals or two meals every other day.

The choice is yours, and whichever path you choose, you'll notice the weight loss process beginning, and you will start to shed those unwanted pounds. By far, IF is the most effective weight loss strategy that exists because it leverages the body's inherent power and unlocks regenerating, calorie-burning, and self-repair mechanisms. Remember, no snacking in between any of the periods! You can have yourself tea or water if you want in between.

I personally eat every other day and keep a 10-hour window and only eat at the frequency of 1 meal, and sometimes two meals per day. I didn't do this

right away, but in incremental steps, as I have previously advised, I worked my way up until I was comfortable to live this lifestyle. What did IF do for me?

It had so many health and wellness benefits. I had better mental clarity and sharpness. I was content, mindful, and self-aware of my eating habits, especially of emotionally triggered eating. I started losing weight rapidly and in a healthy, controlled manner. And best of all, my muscle definition sculpted to the point where I had almost no body fat. I must also advise I exercised rigorously and frequently as well. Exercise, in conjunction with IF is the ultimate combo and guaranteed way to lose weight and transform your body.

Below I have created an outline for you to follow from beginner, intermediate to advanced in regard to eating schedule. Please feel free to modify the schedule to your individual and unique needs as you see fit. Nothing is set in stone; this is a template. But remember no snacking in between any of the periods! Later in this book, I will cover the best choice of food selection, recipes, and personal exercise regimen.

- Beginners IF 6-hour intervals and two meals per day.
- Beginners IF Stage 2 – 8-hour intervals and 2 meals per day
- Beginners IF Stage 3 – 8-hour intervals and 1 meal per day
- Intermediate IF – 10-hour intervals and 1 meal per day
- Intermediate IF stage 2- 12-hour intervals and 1 meal per day
- Advanced IF – 1-day intervals (24 hours) and 1 meal every other day

I have just given you a proven and done for you system that has proof of concept, and that works! This has worked wonders for me and many others too. Now it is up to you to follow and modify the schedule as you see fit, don't begin until you complete the entire book so you can also incorporate the power foods and some delicious recipes. This is your template to success, and all you need to do is follow it, and you should start seeing results anywhere between one to three weeks! Results will vary depending on the level of fasting you select, the foods you choose, and if you exercise too. My advice is to work your way up slowly and measure your progress, and then adjust when you feel comfortable. This is as close as we can get to eating like our ancestors and is what I call functional eating. We eat to survive and not for pleasure; however, if you do decide to have your "cheat meals," just ensure it doesn't dramatically alter your schedule or become habitual.

Our forefathers had some incredible insights into life, and one of them who is world-renowned, Benjamin Franklin, states, "The best of all medicine is resting and fasting." You heard it straight from the horse's mouth and one of the world's greatest inventors who ever lived and walked the face of the planet. He realized something profound that the body inherently possessed its own self-healing, repair mechanisms, and rejuvenating capabilities that don't need to interface with prescription drugs or surgery to attain good health.

This is an incredible truth that one of our forefathers discovered early on, and yet we neglect the power of fasting today, although it has been around since ancient times and the dawn of civilization. Every single major religion worldwide, regardless of belief, ethnicity, race, or creed, all incorporate fasting as part of spiritual enlightenment. This commonality cannot be disputed; we find it among Christians, Hindus, and Buddhists alike who all engage in periods of fasting at different calendar dates for various reasons. Therefore, it should not come to surprise that fasting has so many benefits that range from anti-aging, healing, enhanced cardiovascular and brain functioning, anti-cancer, anti-inflammation, promotes weight loss, improves insulin sensitivity, and strengthens the immune system.

Ultimately, fasting gives your body a well-deserved rest from the foods we are constantly consuming, and our bodies can be thought of as sophisticated pieces of machinery, and just like any machine requires periods of rest or "cooling off time." These periods of rest are essential for us to thrive and to function at optimal capacity.

How (IF) Boosts Our Health?

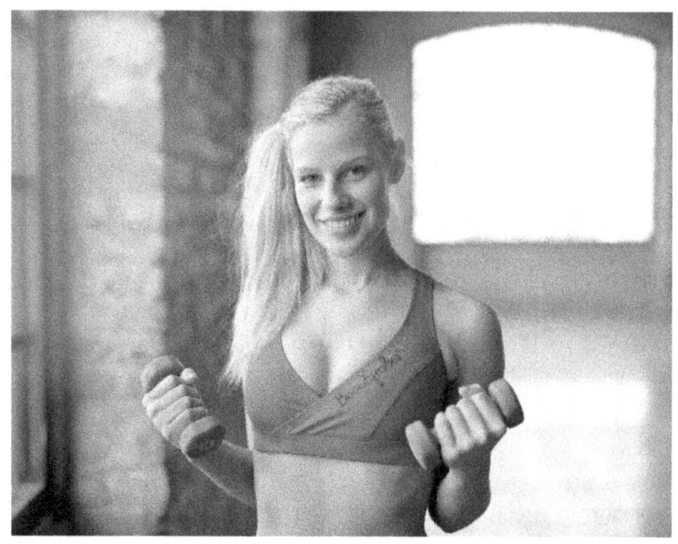

- Diabetes – IF lowers insulin, the fat-storing hormone responsible for excessive weight gain.

- Increases human growth hormone – HGH is responsible for increasing muscle mass, increasing life span, and just making you look better overall.

- Cancer – The number one fueling agent for cancer cells is sugar, and by fasting, you literally starve cells to death, causing "apoptosis," programmed cell death.

- Brain health – People have reported having better mental clarity and sharpness when fasting.
- Anti-Aging – You probably thought over indulging in leafy greens and vegetables was the way to go for anti-aging benefits, right? Well, think again! The elixir of life for anti-aging was right under our noses this whole time! That's right fasting promotes remarkable anti-aging benefits; there is a specific molecule called "beta-hydroxybutyric" that prevents vascular aging within the body. This is the same molecule that activates under the ketogenic diet when the body switches from burning glucose (sugar), which is a primitive form of utilizing energy to using ketones. Basically, sugar burning switching to fat burning.

So, what does this all mean? The use of beta-hydroxybutyric has a chain reaction in the body in specific your DNA, and this change in the body keeps our cells "young" and uncompromised from oxidative stress and free radicals, thus making us immune or less susceptible to chronic degenerative disease states.

High blood pressure – Fasting can reduce high blood pressure due to caloric restriction.

You see, fasting has inherent benefits within our bodies; human beings have evolved over the centuries to eat only when necessary. It wasn't until recently we got exposed to excess eating habits; hence, we lived in a time of scarcity, and food wasn't always readily available like today because of advanced agriculture. Thus, our bodies adapted and conserved energy from foods we ate for extended periods of time. It was normal to go days without food back in the day.

You see, when you stop eating, the hunger hormone called ghrelin gradually decreases in level. Contrary to popular belief, you do not become progressively hungrier as time passes! However, the hunger hormone ghrelin secretes itself in waves of intervals and adapts to your unique eating schedule. Now that's a bit of a mind-bending paradox, and we have all been conditioned to think that if you don't eat, you just become progressively and ferociously hungrier.

A controlled experiment using participants had them go for a 30 hour fast. The results were surprising as when ghrelin levels were measured, and it was observed that ghrelin didn't increase progressively over time, however, but peaked in waves of intervals during the usual eating hours of the participants, and after its peak ghrelin levels decreased and tapered off. Note that the level of the hunger hormones declined even though participants didn't eat anything!

These periods of hunger the participants experienced were consistent with their usual eating hours at breakfast, lunch, and dinner. So, what does this mean for you? This means when you first start to modify your eating habits to reflect IF your feelings of hunger will come and go, and eventually adapt to your new schedule of eating. After a few days, your hormones will adapt to your new eating times, and you will eventually become less and less hungry.

I can tell you that your first week will be the hardest for you to adjust. Remember you spent years developing your habits of eating, but if you stick with the change, your body will adapt.

Mindfulness and Eating

I want to challenge you to really listen to your body the next time you're hungry. I want you to practice mindful eating, from each bite, chew slowly, acknowledge the scent, taste, and even food's sightful appeal, I want you to savor every moment. By doing this, you're really fine-tuning your entire appetite, and you're no longer mindlessly eating, but self-aware and conscious of every meal you have. Often, we find ourselves eating mindlessly, constantly consuming, eating, and eating until we are bloated.

Obviously, being bloated after our meals are not ideal, and thus the importance of mindful eating. Eating excess causes undue hardship to our bodies, which causes more oxidative stress and requires more work for your body to burn calories.

Humans in the 21st century eat for various reasons apart from survival. We no longer just eat functionally, but we eat because of social reasons, emotional, boredom, and flavor. Interestingly enough, when you start practicing mindful eating habits, you'll notice you become satisfied quicker than usual, and it only takes a few bites of food to do so! You may also notice you don't even need to finish your meal, but a few bites and your body is satisfied, hence the importance of really taking the time to listen to how your body responds to certain foods and act accordingly.

If you need flavor in your diet, I suggest incorporating spices or herbs such as salt, oregano, parsley, cayenne pepper, mint, and even lemon juice. This way, your enhancing taste without all the unwanted calories and your ability to satisfy your specific needs.

Lastly, I want to mention relaxing as a strategy while you engage in mindful eating. I know it might sound redundant and obvious, but how many times have you rushed through your meals without giving a second thought to what you are eating? Ingesting whatever is in front of you like there's no tomorrow, so you can make it back to work on time from your lunch break.

There are two nervous systems at work your sympathetic nervous system and parasympathetic nervous system. The sympathetic nervous system is responsible for our fight and flight response and anything "stress" related, so imagine if you're in a rush to finish your meal so you can make it back on time for work to please your boss. You're probably undergoing a certain degree of stress! Thus, you need to seize the moment, plan ahead and take time for yourself to activate the rest and repair nervous system known as the parasympathetic nervous system, which is where resting and healing take place.

If you need flavor in your diet, I suggest incorporating spices or herbs such as salt, oregano, parsley, cayenne pepper, mint, and even lemon juice. This way, your enhancing taste without all the unwanted calories and your ability to satisfy your specific needs.

Lastly, I want to mention relaxing as a strategy while you engage in mindful eating. I know it might sound redundant and obvious, but how many times have you rushed through your meals without giving a second thought to what you are eating? Ingesting whatever is in front of you like there's no tomorrow, so you can make it back to work on time from your lunch break.

There are two nervous systems at work your sympathetic nervous system and parasympathetic nervous system. The sympathetic nervous system is responsible for our fight and flight response and anything "stress" related, so imagine if you're in a rush to finish your meal so you can make it back on time for work to please your boss. - You're probably undergoing a certain degree of stress! Thus, you need to seize the moment, plan ahead and take time for yourself to activate the rest and repair nervous system known as the parasympathetic nervous system, which is where resting and healing take place.

Water and Fiber

Struggling to get full when eating? Why not try incorporating the following simple strategies of increased water and fiber intake? Eat celery or make yourself some celery or vegetable juice, which is an excellent source of fiber that can help you reach a state of satiety. Drink more water with your meals, and don't worry, it won't dilute your digestive acids contrary to popular belief. Water supports your digestive acids as the more water you intake, the more liquid volume you have, which makes the entire digestion process much more efficient and fluid for you.

Salt Deficiency

Sometimes hunger may arise due to the lack of sodium within our diets. Sodium is required for a plethora of physiological functions from inter-cellular communication to the heart functioning and even needed for optimal nerve transmission.

When insulin levels decrease, the more levels of sodium your liver secretes, and hence when you experience bouts of hunger, sometimes it is just your body's way of telling you it is craving some salt. Ergo, when your sodium levels are depleted, the body will release insulin to signal you to replenish sodium supply. Thus, the importance of practicing mindful eating so you can try understanding and fine-tuning your body's specific needs.

Insulin, Glycogen, Glucagon and Fasting

When you eat, insulin normally goes up, and insulin helps you use carbohydrates for energy or stores it as glycogen (deposits of glucose), and when you have too much glycogen stored, the incoming carbs your consuming gets converted into fat. Everything we eat spikes insulin, but at different rates, hence, foods that consist of refined carbohydrates massively spike insulin levels when consumed. After about six hours after you eat, your insulin and blood glucose levels start to diminish, and at this point, your pancreas secretes glucagon, which has an opposite effect on the hormone insulin.

Insulin is responsible for storing energy, but glucagon releases and pulls energy out of your glycogen and fat storage. Another controlled experiment revealed that injecting animals with insulin increased their food consumption, and when animals were injected with glucagon, their food consumption greatly decreased.

Now to tie things all together, have you ever wondered why you never get the feeling of satiety for extended periods of time after eating a bowl of cereal or perhaps pasta? You eat these refined carbs, and then after maybe two hours, you get hungry again. Why does this occur? - This is because when you eat refined foods, your blood sugar and insulin levels elevate rapidly and cause you to be even hungrier! This happens even after all your meals are processed, and there is excess insulin lingering around. The same goes for when you have your mid-night cravings and munch on some snacks or other refined foods, and then when you wake up in the morning, your starving and hungrier than ever before!

Thus, when you are fasting its actual glucagon, that is suppressing your appetite, giving you satiety and burning your stored glycogen and stored fat. There seems to be a common misconception that our brains only run on "glucose," but this is not the case our brain can use ketones for fuel by burning fat. As mentioned earlier, burning sugar for fuel is a more primitive form of utilizing energy our bodies have evolved and are complex and can use fat burning mechanisms too.

Ghrelin and Leptin

So, we know the hormone insulin is tasked with the role of managing blood sugar (glucose) and is responsible for transforming glucose into energy within the intricate and complex systems of our body. But what about the other two hormones are known as "ghrelin" and "leptin"? Which are directly responsible for managing our appetite, ghrelin as previously mentioned is the hunger hormone, and leptin is known as our satiety hormone.

People struggling with obesity tend to have these hormones out of whack. Ghrelin runs rampant within the body, signaling the body to consume more food, and leptin signaling fails to be received, which is responsible for letting you know that you are full of content.

Insulin, ghrelin, and leptin work synergistically, which ultimately helps us complete a whole myriad of bodily functions and essentially determining if we are hungry or not. So, when you are hungry, be aware that the hormone ghrelin is active within your physiology, and vice-versa when your feeling content, the satiety hormone leptin is actively working.

Five Common Cravings

There are typically five major carvings that humans have, which are sweet, salty, sour, spicy, and oily (fats). It is no surprise that food manufacturers leverage these fundamental cravings within our biology to sell their products to us.

The scientist knows if they can trigger our taste buds on our tongue pallet, they can elicit our favorable desires for that particular food product. Being aware of these types of cravings is critical to our health and wellness as well because by understanding and fine-tuning our body's yearnings, we can bring about states of satiety and be content without unhealthily binging on refined foods.

Have you ever tried Keltic sea salt with water? Sometimes it feels so refreshing and rejuvenating as if you have just been recharged, but you'll notice if you continue to drink it, the taste will become rancid. Why does this happen? This is due to the body's need for sodium; hence you start craving salty foods, but once you have replenished your sodium supply anymore salt is excess and unnecessary, ergo the Keltic sea salt drink that was pleasant one moment ago becomes something undesirable. This is simply because our body only needs a certain amount of sodium at a given time, and this principle applies to the other fundamental cravings as well!

Here is the interesting thing, if someone was to put salty chips or perhaps French fries in front of you after you've replenished your sodium supply, and you know this threshold has been reached when the Keltic sea salt drink doesn't taste as appealing to you anymore, guess what?

You probably won't crave the chips or fries because your fundamental salty craving need was met. The human body is an amazing sophisticated piece of biological machinery with many complex intricacies and knows when "enough is enough."

The body knows its daily requirements for essential fats, vitamins, trace minerals and minerals, amino acids, co-factors, and even pro-biotics. The body is an intelligent design and has its own blueprint to function optimally; we just need to provide the right type of raw materials for it to work under its standard operating procedures.

Therefore, whether it's a spicy craving, sour, salty, oily, and even sugar craving, this could just be our bodies signaling us to replenish supplies of certain elements. You can use these strategies to curb any and all of your food cravings!

However, for sugar, I've observed that to curb the sugar cravings, you need to do something different. Simply consuming a banana or apple won't necessarily do the trick for cravings of artificial refined sugars as it is more potent. The best way to tackle this problem is to intake more protein to curb your sugar cravings, you'll notice the more protein you intake, the less you'll crave refined sugars, and ultimately your cravings for something sweet will diminish.

By now, you probably noticed that your "favorite foods" follow the five fundamental cravings all humans have! Is it any wonder why food manufacturers produce their products according to these cravings? If you're going into the food industry business, you can't go wrong with sweet, salty, sour, spicy, and oily foods! – That's why you don't really see bitter or any other type of flavor produced by corporations because they know what your five fundamental cravings are and will only design products to exploit them, they know your weak points.

Everything we've come to know and love in the world of food, donuts, hamburgers, pizza, tacos, and other pastries all use either one element or multiple of our five fundamental cravings!

Foods and Inflammation

You've probably faced some form of inflammation in the past from food you ate, which you had an adverse reaction too? The immune system, which is heavily housed and can be found within your digestive system, is responsible for the defensive response we know as inflammation. The interesting thing about the immune system is that it serves as a duality function meaning the same immune system that heals you from let's say an animal bite wound is the same immune system responsible for heart attacks, joint pain, hives, rashes, redness, headaches, and bodily fatigue.

In this section, I wanted to talk about common foods that can potentially cause you inflammation and is quite contrary to popular belief. Foods that the mainstream media endorses as "healthy foods" when it can actually cause you a lot of harm.

Let's talk about grains, oats, and gluten. I'm sure you have heard about how eating whole grains or oats are good for you by now, and its all the buzz in social media and television, but what if I told you that grains could cause you inflammation! You see, looking at this from an ecological perspective, grains are considered seeds, and nature does not want us eating its seeds. Seeds by design are meant to grow, from seeds sprout apple trees, orange trees, and many other fruit trees.

Since nature doesn't want its seeds eaten as it doesn't serve plants any purpose, thus, these seeds have chemical compounds in them, such as gluten, to serve as a defensive response to being eaten.

Gluten is just one of many plant defense mechanisms that activate when it is consumed. There are other chemical compounds known as phytochemicals called lectin, which is associated with digestive issues, arthritis, and autoimmune diseases. Plants have evolved so much that they can produce a form of "birth control" so animals cannot reproduce their offspring, and these birth control chemicals are known as phytoestrogens.

This is how advanced plants have become they create defensive phytochemicals when consumed in order to cease the reproduction of offspring down the line, so their seeds cannot be eaten. So, you probably think well if I eat gluten-free oats, brownies, pizza, etc. you are going to be alright? Think again. As mentioned earlier, plants have a whole range of inflammation! You see, looking at this from an ecological perspective, grains are considered seeds, and nature does not want us eating its seeds. Seeds by design are meant to grow, from seeds sprout apple trees, orange trees, and many other fruit trees.

Since nature doesn't want its seeds eaten as it doesn't serve plants any purpose, thus, these seeds have chemical compounds in them, such as gluten, to serve as a defensive response to being eaten.

Gluten is just one of many plant defense mechanisms that activate when it is consumed. There are other chemical compounds known as phytochemicals called lectin, which is associated with digestive issues, arthritis, and autoimmune diseases. Plants have evolved so much that they can produce a form of "birth control" so animals cannot reproduce their offspring, and these birth control chemicals are known as phytoestrogens.

This is how advanced plants have become they create defensive phytochemicals when consumed in order to cease the reproduction of offspring down the line, so their seeds cannot be eaten. So, you probably think well if I eat gluten-free oats, brownies, pizza, etc. you're going to be alright? Think again. As mentioned earlier, plants have a whole range of phytochemicals that they use in response to being eaten, and gluten is just one of the many phytochemicals.

But I thought oats were healthy? Yes, they do have healthy nutritional components to them, such as fiber, healthy oils, vitamin E, and protein. But you can think of this as a double-edged sword, and although it has many health benefits, there are potential risks for inflammation.

The best way to figure out if oats or grains affect you is to eat them and observe what happens! Plant seeds want to preserve their survival so they can grow and hence use defensive response chemicals to punish animals or humans for deciding to eat them.

Socially Engineered to Constantly Eat – Corporations and Their Vested Interest

In my introduction, I briefly touched on how animals in the wild don't eat out of boredom, but out of necessity to survive. I painted you the example of the content lion whom we consider the king of the jungle and a ferocious beast. However, interestingly enough, when even these majestic creatures are content, they do no hunt for prey to eat.

So, who came up with this whole notion to constantly be eating at almost every part of our day? We are bombarded constantly with commercials from McDonald's, KFC, Burger King, etc. and the motive behind these marketing tactics is to take your money! You see corporations behind all the fast-food chains and the entire food empire per se have their own vested interests to sell to you, and it is certainly not for your benefit. They have ulterior motives and could care less about your health and wellness!

I want you to think critically who designed this framework of eating breakfast, lunch, and dinner, and of course, "snacking" in-between with more junk food? Breakfast, lunch, and dinner have been commercialized so much to condition us that we don't even question it! -It is just a normal part of life going through the drive-thru of McDonald's to get our fix. Corporations are the most anti-human entities on the planet. They could care less about your health and wellness. Did you know fast-food franchises, and as a matter of fact, the entire food empire hires food scientists to do their "dirty work"? What do I mean by this?

Well, you see food scientist is hired to design and manufacture foods that are addictive to you and me. That's right, I said addictive, the same kind of addiction drug addicts have is essentially the same results they try to emulate from us too and is it any coincidence that the primary go-to ingredient for almost all food additives is some form of sugar!

That's right, and I said sugar! I am not talking about the kind of sugar our body uses for fuel (glucose), although excess amounts can be harmful as previously discussed; however, I am specifically talking about refined and processed sugar that food manufacturers incorporate into all their products.

There are actually different types of sugars, and corporations have become sneaky and have concealed the generally known term of sugar by using other forms, substitutes, or sweeteners.

We need to become proficient label deck readers in order to understand the kinds of foods we are eating. But a general rule of thumb to keep you safe is anything found at the supermarket that can be bought in a cardboard box and has an extended shelf-life should be considered harmful to your health.

Now let's go over the different forms of sugar and artificial sweeteners that you may not be able to easily recognize at first glance.

Six Types of Sugars to Lookout For

- Dextrose

- Fructose

- Sucrose

- Maltose

- Lactose

- Galactose

Artificial Sweeteners to Lookout For

- Saccharin

- Aspartame

- Corn Syrup

- Advantame

- Neotame

- Stevia

- Acesulfame

Substitute for Sugars to Lookout for

- Molasses

- Honey

- Xylitol

- Brown rice syrup

- Coconut palm sugar

- Date sugar

- Maple Syrup

- Agave Syrup

- Brown rice Syrup

- Coconut Palm Sugar

We need to become aware of the many hidden forms of sugar food manufacturing corporations sneak into our foods. Hence, the importance of becoming a proficient ingredient deck label reader!

A statistic revealed that the average American eats excessive amounts of 200,000 lbs. of sugar every single year! The fact is we only need a tablespoon of sugar (natural) within our bloodstream at any given point in time. Sugar can be a dangerous substance and has volatile characteristics, and simply put, it can make things explode literally!

You see, because sugar can be explosive, our bodies have evolved to develop complex mechanisms and procedures to store sugar efficiently. Due to the explosive nature of sugar, the hormones insulin facilitates the transferring of excess sugar to fat, and hence why we see refined sugar being the primary cause of weight gain in North America.

Sugar Addiction

Sugar addiction is a real thing as strange as it may sound people have addictions to sugar! Corporations have exploited this drive we all possess inherently and the craving for something sweet, which elicits feelings of euphoria. Corporations go to the extreme in order to get us hooked they actually do lab experiments on people by having them enter the MRI while eating a particular food that can be a chocolate bar, chips, etc. and what this does is it reveals brain activity through the MRI, and scientist use this information to craft food products insidiously.

Our brains light up at certain regions which correspond to the stimulus consumed (food) and scientist take a close look at the regions that have been stimulated and design their food products accordingly.

You'd probably be surprised to know that usually, all these mega food franchises like McDonald's, Harveys, Subway, Burger King, Dunkin' Donuts, and many more companies share the same supplier that provides them carefully crafted and specifically designed food products that have addictive properties. Some sort of food manufacturing plant that has food-scientist working for them to create the "secrete" or ideal recipes that make these companies their fortune. – Sounds like something out of science fiction, right? But the sad truth is this is far from fiction and is the reality we live in.

There was a scientific study conducted by the University of Bordeaux in France by Dr. Serge Ahmed, who was using rats in a controlled experiment, and this experiment entailed sugar and cocaine as the stimulus. Both researchers and Dr. Serge were surprised at the outcome of this experiment because the rats were given both cocaine and sugar, and they wanted to know which was the preferred stimulus. To their shock, the rats actually choose sugar over cocaine! -That's right; they choose refined sugar over the notorious drug cocaine.

The study revealed the addictive powers of sugar and why it's a substance to be leery of and something to be avoided. This explains a lot actually if you really come to think about it? We see in this modern-day people who cannot control their eating habits or should I say binge eating habits when it comes to refined sugar. I have a challenge for you, or perhaps this is something you can be made aware of if you think back. Have you ever tried an Oreo cookie, chips, maybe Doritos, or your favorite pack of donuts? Can you honestly tell me that you've only stopped eating one? Truthfully, you most likely demolished the whole box!

The simple fact is you couldn't control yourself to the addictive appeal of sugar! " It just tastes so darn good," sweet yet addictive and harmful to your well-being, eliciting feelings of bliss and euphoria, and let's not forget responsible for the degeneration of health and the catalyst to many chronic degenerative diseases when you have constant exposure to it over time.

The issue here is humans have mastered the craft of manipulating almost anything into specific concentrations; for instance, heroin comes from poppy seeds, cocaine from cocoa plants, and alcohol from grains. In their natural forms, these plant components are quite harmless; however, when precisely extracted into concentrations is where the trouble arises. These are naturally occurring substances we get from our planet, but through devious manipulation techniques and procedures, these pristine substances produce addictive compounds!

Food manufacturing corporations and scientist probably have a laugh saying " I dare you to try just one", and I'm sure this is probably a slogan that a food company probably used in their marketing camping at some point in time, however, they know deep down inside they are manipulating our biology and exploiting our built-in drives to create habitual forming products that are engineered to be simply irresistible!

The industrialization and advance agriculture of our society wherein lies the problem, when we refine these substances in their most concentrated form to get you hooked and is where the addiction and misery of many people over the century was born.

Historical Corporate Use of Addictive Substances

Coca-Cola, arguably the world's most successful soft drink brand that came into existence in the late 19th century, has used questionable substances in the past that gave "coke" its addictive quality. Even this big brand name has some skeletons in the closet. Did you know in the early 1900s, Coca-Cola actually had trace amounts of cocaine in it?! Yes, this is not a myth, but the truth is Coca-Cola used cocaine in specific concentrations in varying amounts, which most likely gave "coke" its addictive hook. It must be noted that cocaine was legal at the time during the periods of 1886 –

1929 and was used for medicinal purposes, and cocaine is still used today for medical purposes.

But eventually, the government regulatory bodies caught up and prohibited the use of cocaine publicly, especially in food. Thus, cocaine was outlawed, and Coca-Cola had to find a new addictive ingredient, and they turned to refined sugar and caffeine, which is still used to this day.

I don't think I have to go into detail of why caffeine is addictive, as well. I'm pretty sure you know by now, this substance also contains habitual forming addictive properties and is used by all fast food restaurant chains worldwide when they're serving you your "morning fix."

SLIP

Have you heard of the term SLIP? This is the terminology used by food scientists and describes the phenomenon of the rate at which food slips down your throat. Fast food manufacturers are privy to this information and exploit it because they know our human biology, and the faster food slips down our throat, the more we will potentially eat. Why is this?

When we eat normally, we chew our foods into a mushy paste before swallowing, and this also prepares our digestive enzymes, and other

biochemical processes within our body and food manufacturers know that this requires a lot of energy, thus they try to trick our bodies by expediting the journey of food and making it travel down our digestive system faster so that way we can continue to eat more! -They understand that the more we chew foods, specifically foods that are natural (whole foods), the more work is required for our bodies to utilize energy, and thus the less food we will eat.

Ergo, refining foods is to their advantage as they have been stripped bare and have little to no fiber or nutrition, hence why we can consume loads of refined foods in a single sitting versus eating whole foods that fill us up much faster with much less.

As you can see, the people, or should I say corporations behind all the big food brands that you crave, have figured us all out. They have been deconstructing our basic and fundamental human biology and exploiting our biochemistry to push their irresistible products to us so they can make a fortune. They are literally pushing our buttons and manipulating us through flavor and other appealing features. You may argue well, and we have free choice or free moral agency to do whatever we choose; however, you must understand that there is a toxic miasma present, and food manufacturers are exploiting our very biology in order to control us. When is the last time you had only one Oreo cookie or ate one piece of the chip from your favorite junk food brand? - The answer is most likely never! This is because it's almost as if we don't have a choice but to eat their food via the manipulation of our senses.

Therefore, it is so important to be aware and follow my strategies in order to be liberated from this food empire's tyranny. We need to understand intermittent fasting, mindful eating, and the power of whole foods, which I will discuss later in this book, and the consequences of eating "Frankenstein foods." These substances used in our modern-day food supply are habit forming, and thus keep us coming back for more and more with dire consequences to our health that corporations could care less about!

Even from the way foods are packaged, designed, and boxed have all been scientifically proven to captivate us and thus make us purchase their product. Next time you go to McDonald's, I want you to observe how the packaging is, and soon you'll notice similarities to how opening up that big mac that has been wrapped up for you is likened to opening Christmas gifts!

What do I mean by this? Food manufacturers have studied the psychology behind us, what makes us tick, what makes us happy, and ultimately why we desire things. They know the psychology behind our buying habits so much that they even understand emulating "gift-wrap" for Christmas creates a sense of excitement and joy sub-consciously when we are unwrapping our foods from the wrapper. They know by subtly exploiting our sub-conscious drives as well they can enhance our experience when we participate in their products. Hence the importance of being aware of these things and reverse hacking the exploits they have put us under.

Intermittent Fasting – The Best Anti- Aging Strategy

Earlier in this book, I mentioned anti-aging is one of the many benefits of IF. If we break IF down at its most fundamental level, we are essentially looking at "caloric restriction," which simply put is restricting the calories you consume. Besides, who do you think came up with the notion of constantly eating throughout the day? – I can give you a hint it starts with a "c," and I am sure you guessed by now if you guessed corporations your absolutely right! Of course, corporations want you eating more its in their vested interest that you are eating their products throughout the day. They want you to buy more and more and could care less about you as an individual; however, they're more concerned with making money.

This is a vicious cycle if you look at it from the outside, imagine this, you eat poorly, and as a result, you have poor health, and you have to go to the doctors for medical intervention for whatever disease you're stuck with because of your poor food choices. The result is both physical and financial misery and what a terrible way to live life! – But by the end of this book, I hope you will break this vicious cycle!

Caloric restriction is not complicated at all! The less you eat, the less load or less work is required from your body. The more work our bodies are subject too, the faster we age, and thus the higher the chance of susceptibility to chronic diseases. The more metabolic work our body is involved with, the shorter our lifespan will be, and a controlled study conducted with lab animals proves this point. There were two groups of mice group A and group B, group A was given the standard diet, but group B was denied food and put under caloric restriction. In short, group B lived significantly longer than their counterparts and lived healthier!

Group A's lifespan was cut much shorter, and they seemed to acquire chronic diseases much more easily. Case in point the power of caloric restriction for anti-aging and longevity.

I hear misinformation left, right, and center, and one time on T.V I heard a supposed fitness "expert," claiming that we should raise our metabolism. First off, I want to tell you this is a terrible idea and raising your metabolism will do nothing good for your health-wise. We should have our metabolic rate strong, stable, and slow, not fast. Our metabolism can be defined as the sum total of all our bodily chemical reactions, both chemicals that build up our body and break down our body.

Did you know animals that live shorter lives have faster metabolisms? And animals that live long have slow and steady metabolisms. You see, the more energy the body spends on digestion, absorption, and processing foods, the less energy it will have to spend on anti-aging, building muscle, and both growth and repair functions. As you can see, eating more is a disservice to our bodies and causes a lot more harm than good. On top of that, interestingly enough, when our bodies run low on energy, this is when the emergency response system kicks in, and we run into some serious problems.

The point is you don't want to raise your metabolism; however, you want to re-allocate where energy is spent within your metabolism and balance things out that is the key. It doesn't matter if your only eating healthy too, whether its salad, lean meat, etc. this is all still considered work for the body! Digestion, absorption, allocating energy, and expelling waste all require your body to work.

Just like any machine, the body needs rest too. So, what happens if you don't give your body the deserved rest it requires? Remember earlier, and I mentioned if your body runs low on energy meaning your constantly eating not giving it any rest, then this is when the emergency response kicks in. It's sort of like having too many applications working on your computer, and the system is overwhelmed and freezes, and then your forced to go into "safe mode," and in this mode, you can only use your computer at its most basic functions and features. In this same way, when you're constantly eating and forcing your body to work 24/7 365 days year-round, your body will not perform at its optimal potential.

Just like how you need to go on vacation from work every now and then, your body also needs to go on "holiday" from eating too. You see, when you take a break from food, your body can now use its precious resources on things like repair, healing, strengthening, growth, and anti-aging because energy can be redistributed into these avenues. – The whole digestion process is a lot of work. Do you ever get sleepy after a big meal? Well, that's because digestion is extremely taxing on the body.

Now you can see why eating 5-6 meals a day is a very bad idea, and so is messing with your metabolism. Some people and even dietitians have this misinformed concept that eating food all day like how cows graze on grass all day is good for you, but they are sadly mistaken.

Cows have four stomachs, while humans only have one!

Diabetes and Fasting

Earlier in this chapter, I touched briefly and discussed the hormone insulin and its relation to glycogen and glucagon. I want to elaborate further on the role of insulin and its connection to diabetes, and also how fasting can drastically improve and even reverse this chronic condition.

I mentioned when you eat anything, insulin is up-regulated, meaning its actively working and is responsible for telling cells when to divide, grow, and manage blood sugar levels. Now imagine if you're constantly eating, which is the primary stimulus for insulin secretion, the body eventually becomes numb to insulin due to overexposure, and hence you get something called insulin sensitivity, which is the hallmark of type 2 diabetes.

Cells become resistant and stop listening. This is when a plethora of problems arise; heart, blood pressure, brain, auto-immune disease, and inflammation all stem from insulin resistance, and doctors have coined this fancy term as a metabolic syndrome, which basically means your whole body is out of whack or messed up.

Fasting just a few days can help revitalize your body's response to insulin. Having insulin resistance only prolongs your overweight problem as you'll start to store more fat in your cells as opposed to burning them. The thing is, although your body becomes unresponsive to insulin in regard to cell feeding, however, the body will continue storing fat continuously, and this is why we see a lot of the times generally speaking people with diabetes tend to have weight issues.

Hence, the importance of fasting cannot be understated. As soon as you start to fast, you will see that metabolic syndrome symptoms start to disappear and eventually reverse. Your diabetes won't heal overnight but will take time and with the right nutritional protocol alongside with IF you will be able to regain your health.

Exercise and Intermittent Fasting

Whether your bodybuilding or just trying to get in shape, IF enhances your body capacity to build muscle! When you start to fast between one to two days between workout periods, genes called sirtuins activate, which are linked anti-aging and muscle building.

I'm sure you heard about how resting is as important as weight lifting when it comes to gaining muscle, and much is the same as the principle of fasting. Your body needs rest from the constant processing of food and the many biochemical procedures required, and by doing so, the body can redistribute energy to other departments such as bodybuilding, fat burning, repair, and growth.

Not All Calories Weight-loss Strategies Are Equal

You hear a lot of dietitians, and even doctors talk about calories but never really make the distinction between empty calories and dense calories full of nutrition. This is a big disservice to the general public as this misleads the masses to assume that all calories are equal, which is not the case. Not all calories are made equal!

Refined and processed foods contain mostly empty calories. Remember, these foods have been stripped of their nutrients, minerals, and vitamins; perhaps at best, they have some sort of additive like fiber to enhance the product, but nonetheless, overall, it's still junk food. Whole foods, on the other hand, are calorie dense-packed with essential nutrients, fats, fiber, and other trace minerals that your body requires to function optimally.

This is a distinction that you must be made aware of because many people are misled to believe eating calories from a baked pizza is the same as calories from a healthy salad bowl. Calories are not all the same, thus be cognizant of the type of calorie your eating, especially if your one to measure your daily caloric intake.

Don't Use Willpower to Fast

I'm a firm believer in willpower when it comes to pursuing your dreams, ambition, and fulfilling your goals in life. However, when it comes to built-in hard-wired human drives, I am not so much a big advocate when it comes to fasting and consuming foods. Now, this might sound puzzling or quite paradoxical because your thinking you need to have a certain measure of willpower to abstain from junk foods, and you are probably right to a certain degree you do need resolve and determination to refrain from unhealthy foods.

But I am a firm believer in promoting satiety over willpower, and by this, we are hacking into our internal base drives at the most fundamental and instinctive levels. Think about it we are up against corporations who have been exploiting our built-in drives for over centuries now, and thus it would make sense for us to fight back by "flipping the script" and reverse engineering what they've done to us.

How do we do this? Consume a diet rich in whole foods, protein, coconut oils, meats, and healthy fats! I will go into more detail about this later in the book, but that is basically the gist of it. Finding ways to curb our cravings for refined foods by replacing them with foods that can meet our built-in drives.

Willpower alone is useless, and I wouldn't recommend solely relying on willpower for fasting. As mentioned before, your first week of IF will probably be your hardest, but once you have broken into it, you will start to get the hang of it and understand your body in a deeper and intimate way. You'll be able to start fine-tuning your needs and truly understand hunger.

But I am a firm believer in promoting satiety over willpower, and by this, we are hacking into our internal base drives at the most fundamental and instinctive levels. Think about it we are up against corporations who have been exploiting our built-in drives for over centuries now, and thus it would make sense for us to fight back by "flipping the script" and reverse engineering what they've done to us.

How do we do this? Consume a diet rich in whole foods, protein, coconut oils, meats, and healthy fats! I will go into more detail about this later in the book, but that is basically the gist of it. Finding ways to curb our cravings for refined foods by replacing them with foods that can meet our built-in drives.

Willpower alone is useless, and I wouldn't recommend solely relying on willpower for fasting. As mentioned before, your first week of IF will probably be your hardest, but once you have broken into it, you will start to get the hang of it and understand your body in a deeper and intimate way. You'll be able to start fine-tuning your needs and truly understand hunger.

A lot of the time, when we eat, we are not actually hungry but have been programmed by society to eat. You'll notice when you start fasting, there is a distinct difference between psychological eating and physiological eating. When you eat, it is due psychologically to social conditioning and not the true need to eat, but when you eat physiologically, it's for functionality and the need to survive like the animals in the wild.

Remember, I am not asking you to starve yourself but to take extended periods of time or windows and fast. Don't jump into its cold turkey but follow my instructions and incrementally build your way up to your comfort level. The truth is everybody should fast as a health protocol and benefit, not enough of us do and suffer from many health problems consequently. Once you've become accustomed to IF you'll realize that your "old hunger" becomes more of a mental sensation than a physical need.

I don't believe in using willpower to control our built-in drives; however, we need to learn how to manage and guide our cravings by using nutritional strategies.

Things to Consider

Many diets propose a one size fits all method and this is inherently wrong and contains many erroneous principles behind it. We know every individual is unique and will need a specialized approach and diet plan designed for their specific needs. Earlier, I discussed the five fundamental cravings, and each person has his or her own preferred desirable taste. Every individual will like one taste appeal over the other.

However, when it comes to fasting, everyone benefits from it regardless of age. But the only exception is the intensity of the fast as each person is equipped to handle IF at different levels as we are all unique and have different physiological needs and capacities.

Have you ever watched the show "Biggest Loser" I'm sure you've heard of this program on T.V before? Contestants who are obese go on the show and take on a challenge to lose weight within a certain set period of time. A big component not publicized enough apart from diet modifications like the ketogenic or low carb diet - fasting is at the forefront and aids participants in losing large amounts of weight. Simply put, they restrict calories and utilize IF.

But, interestingly enough, you never really hear from the participants again after their showtime run finishes. On other reality shows, there is usually some sort of "reunion" type of theme, but in this case, we don't really see that. One should also note that participants do sign a nondisclosure agreement, which makes sense why we don't really hear much from them.

Now, what point am I trying to get across? Well, did you know a good amount of these contestants lose weight successfully, but after a short period of time, gain it all back!

To understand this, we must dig deeper and understand what happens to us when we eat. So, we know when we eat, insulin is secreted in varying amounts, and sugar and fat are stored in the liver. But when too much incoming sugar appears, your body starts to convert and store fat in excess amounts.

There is this flawed notion, and I'm pretty sure you've heard this popular phrase "calories in and calories out," which is very flawed. As explained earlier, not all calories are made equal, and depending on various factors, including biochemistry and what type of calories you consume will dictate if it is stored or burned. So, what happens when you have insulin insensitivity? Does your body burn fat as effectively according to the calorie in calorie out model? Absolutely not, because without insulin delegating storing and fat burning you will not be able to access the fat burning mechanisms due to the lack of responsiveness of insulin, hence the importance of "re-sensitizing" your insulin hormone through IF.

This is why we see so many contestants fail in the long run because they are simply following a flawed system and model that simply does not work. Neglecting the whole picture and ignoring the crucial master hormone insulin does people a disservice, and now we can see why these contestants gain back all their weight.

There is this popular myth out there about if you fast, you are going to "burn muscle," and I can tell you this is false. Studies confirm this that your protein is preserved and stays intact as oppose to being burned, as many mistakenly think. Rest assure IF will not burn lean muscle; however, it is possible you may not build as fast or become as "big" due to the lack of protein intake. But, overall, IF will enhance muscle building and repair processes.

Different Forms of Fasting

There are different types or forms of fasting that you can try. Ideally, the cessation of all food consumption is the best type of fast, but if you want, when starting out, you can try the following types of fasts to get you familiar with the process. Then you can slowly work your way up to higher-level fasts mentioned in the book in incremental steps.

Types of Fast

- Fruit Juice fast
- Vegetable juice fast
- Smoothie fast
- Water fasts

Why Intermittent Fasting Is a Foolproof Strategy

The ultimate detox, cleanse, and universally accessible weight-loss method is intermittent fasting! Anybody can do it! People of all ages, whether male or female it doesn't matter. There is absolutely no reason why you cannot start IF today! It is completely free, so what is your excuse?

Think about it with intermittent fasting. You don't have to shop, clean, or even meal prep anything! Whether your vegan, don't eat meat, have nut allergies, don't have money, or travel, the bottom line is you can still fast!

Advantages of Intermittent Fasting:

- Simple
- Free
- Accessible
- Healthy
- Convenient
- Flexible
- Start anytime
- No restrictions
- Safe (Preferably under medical supervision)
- Allows the body to rest
- Enables growth, repair, and regenerative capacities
- Helps with muscle preservation and definition
- Cleanses and detox Body
- Restores balance
- Longevity and increased life span
- Anti-aging benefits

It is incredible that such a simple yet profound technique that has been known since ancient times can be used to improve your health from a holistic standpoint. Remember, our bodies are like machines, and thus we need to take special care of this sophisticated piece of machinery we have been blessed with, and you can start improving your health and losing weight simply by fasting!

Bariatric Surgery - Gastric Sleeve and Gastric By-Pass

If you have ever considered getting a gastric sleeve done, which is also known as "bariatric surgery," I want to give you the facts and my take on surgery for weight loss. Surgery for weight loss can be effective, but it is NOT something I recommend to anyone! I don't really see it as a health-promoting effort nor something long term without complications.

So, what exactly is a gastric sleeve? Well, doctors literally cut up your stomach and resize it to 15% of its original size and use medical grade staples to close the incisions. A gastric by-pass, which is also a medical procedure, is when a surgeon divides your stomach into smaller upper pouches, which are rearranged to connect to your small intestine. There are many variations of this medical procedure.

Now I am just appalled that this is even a remotely available option here in the 21st century, nothing can be more barbaric than having someone go inside your body, cut, solder, and rearrange your organs in order to help you lose weight. Is it just me that thinks that this is a little insane? – Of course, the procedure works effectively, but what they don't tell you is the long-term complications that come with it!

In theory, it sounds good that by reducing the size of your stomach, you also thereby decrease appetite and your capacity to eat. But let's look at some of the complications and risks associated with bariatric surgery that aren't highlighted or nearly emphasized enough!

Complications and Risks to Bariatric Surgery:

- Bowel obstructions
- Loss of urinary control
- Puking and Vomiting
- Bleeding
- Gall bladder rupture
- Fatigue
- Ulcers
- Depression from other side effects
- Nausea
- Painful digestion
- Inability to control defecating

These are only a small list of complications and side effects that you will experience after surgery, and there are many more. You can expect frequent visits to the hospital due to all the complications, but what do you expect you allowed a surgeon to go inside of you and literally butcher your organs!

I wrote this book to save you from going down this road and let you know that there are other alternatives that are much safer, effective, and healthier than going in for surgery. Please, I admonish you and even beg you to listen to my advice as you will have regret going down the path of weight loss surgery. I have met many people who have had this procedure done, and they all regret it! -It really is a short-lived experience, and while you may rapidly lose weight initially, but you will be living with long term health complications that will seriously affect your quality of life.

Not only is it a physical burden but also a financial one too. The surgery itself is quite expensive, and you may get lucky enough to have insurance cover it, but I can tell you that there will be even bigger expenses down the road due to the complications that the surgery brings. It is not natural for the body to be cut open and have its organs removed, resized or even rearranged.

There is this propaganda being fed to the masses and that it is in your genes to be "fat" or overweight. Who do you think this serves? Definitely not you, but the agenda of corporations, and you can see an almost symbiotic relationship with food corporations are producing foods that cause diseases including obesity, and then hospitals are having to treat you for your ailments. It's a vicious cycle and an extremely profitable business model. It is almost as if food manufactures and the modern medical system are in collusion together!

This so anti-human on so many levels. What benefit does this really serve you except a series of unfortunate events that will unfold due to you putting your trust in the medical model? Remember, your battle is with addictive and habitual forming foods that use substances that exploit our built-in drives. Genes are secondary to lifestyle and environmental influences, meaning your genes turn on and off like lights and are secondary to the decisions you make and what you expose yourself too.

Although genes contain the blueprint and play an integral role in determining certain physical attributes or the expression of them, however, genes alone don't cause obesity! Imagine a plane crash, do we blame gravity for this? Certainly not, although gravity is fundamental and so our genes, but the direct cause and effect cannot originate from gravity alone. But the events preceding the plane crash, such as human error, mechanical issues, terrorism, or even weather. Do you understand now why genes are secondary?

The human body is an intelligent design and is so sophisticated that it knows what it needs. Possess renewing, regenerating capabilities, and self-healing mechanisms that are inherently found within everyone's body! This is a divine gift that everyone possess and has access too. The key is to learn how to leverage this healing system, and that is through proper nutrition, exercise, and fasting!

Any doctor telling you to go the route of bariatric surgery needs to be fired! – And held accountable. Without even touching on other alternative health strategies that work, and to solely have you go down this path for their financial gain is a crime to humanity. So why isn't fasting endorsed by the medical professionals that we hold on a pedestal?

Because there is no money! That's right, no financial gain! What would it profit the medical system to endorse fasting? They wouldn't be able to make money off telling you a strategy that is completely free, non-invasive, safe, and even more effective than weight loss surgery. This is the world we are living in, and that's why it is incredibly important to become self-aware. The purpose of this entire book is to give you the truth and nothing but the truth, and of course, holistic strategies you can use for weight loss.

Fasting has proven time and time again that it is the ultimate weight loss strategy that exists from even ancient times. Doctors know this but seem only to promote their own agenda.

Thus, if you have ever considered bariatric surgery, please take the time to reconsider and really analyze the facts and weigh the risks versus the outcome. It is not worth doing as its really a short cut, and all short cuts come with immense repercussions.

You will lose weight through IF, but you just need to take action, stick with the program, and trust the process.

Summary of Intermittent Fasting

You've reached the end of this chapter, and I would like to give you a small recap of what you learned. IF has existed since ancient times and has been observed to elicit immense health benefits ranging from weight loss, repair and growth, regeneration, and healing. Below are terms I would like to clarify in case you may have gotten confused and note I provide you a glossary at the end of the book for definitions.

Intermittent fasting – Periodic fasting at any given period of time. Eight hours, 6 hours, 12 hours, or even 24-hour windows before you eat.

Calories restriction – Eating less food or consuming fewer calories by eating less food.

Fasting – Refraining from consuming food.

The distinction between hunger for functional eating and hunger for habitual or psychosocial eating must be known. You must be aware of the mind and body disconnect because only then you can truly understand if you are truly hungry or not.

Hence, the importance of mindful eating and becoming aware, fine-tuning your body's physiological needs versus psychological wants. Your mind can be your greatest ally or foe, depending on how you condition it! Meaning if you let your mind take control and allow it to dictate your eating behavior based on craving substances that exploit our built-in drives, then you will surely lose the battle.

But if you focus and listen to what your body is telling you and practice functional eating like animals in the wild, you will come on top every time. Remember, there are various hormones at play when eating and fasting, but the three major hormones at the forefront are insulin, ghrelin, and leptin.

Ghrelin is responsible for the feeling of hunger and is released in waves of intervals and does not progressively build up contrary to popular belief. Leptin is responsible for satiety, and leveraging this hormone is essential to achieve states of contentment. Insulin is considered a master hormone of sorts and is responsible for delegating sugar and fat burning and storage, and as well as many more functions.

Like insulin resistance, leptin resistance is a phenomenon that occurs within people who struggle with excess weight. Leptin tells you to stop eating, but we see some people are unresponsive to leptin and thus don't get the "I'm satisfied" signal and continue to consume more food than required. Thus, not only does IF re-sensitizes your response to insulin, but it also re-sensitizes your response to leptin, thereby helping you feel satisfied when you eat again.

You can think of it as a full-body reset, just like how you reset your computer when multiple browsers are open, causing you to lag.

Once you're in a state of fasting, your body now can focus and allocate its precious resources to healing, growth, and repair mechanisms, and no longer divert energy to processing foods via digestion. Basically, your body gets to do some much-needed maintenance or "spring cleaning" when you fast.

Like insulin resistance, leptin resistance is a phenomenon that occurs within people who struggle with excess weight. Leptin tells you to stop eating, but we see some people are unresponsive to leptin and thus don't get the "I'm satisfied" signal and continue to consume more food than required. Thus, not only does IF re-sensitizes your response to insulin, but it also re-sensitizes your response to leptin, thereby helping you feel satisfied when you eat again.

You can think of it as a full-body reset, just like how you reset your computer when multiple browsers are open, causing you to lag.

Once you're in a state of fasting, your body now can focus and allocate its precious resources to healing, growth, and repair mechanisms, and no longer divert energy to processing foods via digestion. Basically, your body gets to do some much-needed maintenance or "spring cleaning" when you fast.

The incredible benefits of IF cannot be emphasized enough. Through fasting, you can relief auto-immune diseases temporarily, reduce seizures, lowers cholesterol, revitalizes skin, sharpens your alertness, and much, much more!

Warnings to Consider

Before starting any new regiments, please consult your doctor or licensed health care professional and see if there may be any risks or health complications associated with IF due to your current circumstances.

Also, if you are struggling with high levels of insulin, low blood sugar levels may cause migraines, therefore consult your doctor and ask how you can incorporate a modified IF to your lifestyle.

Chapter 2: Precautions During Intermittent Fasting

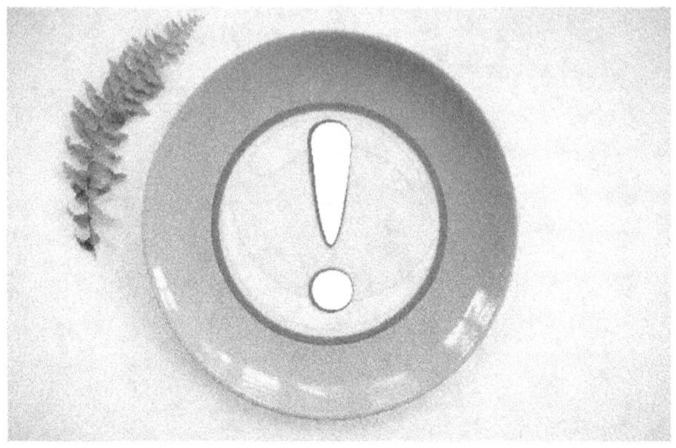

Although intermittent fasting may seem like an ideal diet plan for those who want to lose their weight or improve their health, you ought to choose the best diet plan for you. You should note that intermittent fasting has some advantages and disadvantages, before getting to know which precautions you should take note of while fasting.

Advantages of Intermittent Fasting

Intermittent fasting has incredible benefits not only to women's body and brain but also to men's. The following are a few of the benefits linked to intermittent starvation:

Altering the functioning of body cells and hormones: Intermittent fasting practiced for a while brings several alterations in your body. For your body to make more fats accessible, it tends to initiate significant cell repair processes and also changes the levels of hormones in your body. The levels of insulin in your body drop, facilitating the breakdown of fats. Growth hormones also increase as the blood levels in them increase a factor that facilitates muscle gaining. The body induces processes such as cellular repairing and removal of any waste materials from the cells.

Lose of weight and belly calories: Intermittent fasting is done to lose weight as you only take in a few meals. Intermittent fasting enhances your metabolic rate, which helps your body burn excess fats such as the belly fats. Studies show that intermittent fasting leads to a 3-8 percent weight loss if done for around three to twenty-four weeks. Observation shows that within this fasting duration, four to seven percent of people lost their belly fats, one of the toxic fats in a human's body responsible for various illnesses.

Reduces the resistance of insulin:

Intermittent fasting reduces the insulin levels in your body that, in turn, lowers risks of Type 2 Diabetes, which has been a common illness. The common characteristics of diabetes include high levels of blood sugar in the situation of insulin battle. Thus, intermittent fasting helps in lowering the levels of insulin, which helps in preventing this illness. It also helps protect any possible damages that can affect your kidneys.

Reduction of oxidative constant worry and body inflammation: Intermittent fasting helps reduce stress, which is one of the riskiest ways of fast aging as well as other chronic illnesses. Free radicals are the molecules responsible for reacting with molecules such as DNA and proteins and destroy them. Intermittent fasting, therefore, helps fight body inflammation and destroy any molecules responsible for constant worries.

Heart health: Intermittent fasting is beneficial for your heart's health and prevents you from any heart diseases. Since it regulates sugar levels in your body, intermittent fasting prevents you from high blood pressure, and inflammatory markers, and cholesterol levels hence maintaining heart health.

Induction of cellular restoration procedures: When you fast, your body initiates the cell's 'waste elimination' procedures that are known as autophagy. Body cells break down and metabolize the dysfunctional proteins that accumulate inside the body cells. Increased waste elimination prevents your body against other illnesses such as Alzheimer's disease, one of the common neurodegenerative disorders with no cure.

Prevention against cancer: After your body eliminates any dysfunctional cells that accumulate over time, your body becomes free from any cancer risks. The uncontrolled development of cells is one of the common characteristics of cancer, and therefore, intermittent fasting facilitates your body's metabolic rate, which helps reduce any possible risks of cancer. Intermittent fasting also reduces several impacts of chemotherapy.

Brain health: Since intermittent fasting is better for your body, then it is best for your brain. Reduction of oxidative stress and various worries is advantageous for your brain fitness. Recurrent fasting increases the development of new nerves, which improves the functioning of your brain. It also helps in increasing brain hormone levels known as the Brain-derived neurotropic factors, which helps fight depression and any other brain-related illnesses. Intermittent fasting also helps fight brain damages caused by stroke.

Extending lifespan: Intermittent fasting can help you live longer due to its ability to control metabolism rates, regulating blood sugar levels, and eliminating any dysfunctional cells within your body.

Disadvantages of Intermittent Fasting

Unfortunately, intermittent fasting has cons, too, especially to the females. Studies show that before trying intermittent fasting, you should always contact your physician. The following are the disadvantages associated with intermittent fasting:

It is not risk-free: Intermittent fasting is not advisable to people who are at higher health risks such as those over sixty-five years. People under medical conditions, high fat needs, the diabetic, the underweight, the underage, pregnant, and those breastfeeding cannot undertake intermittent fasting.

You will be hungry: During intermittent fasting, you might have a grumbling stomach, especially if you have correctly been observing the correct dietary plans. You should avoid looking at, smelling, or even thinking about food while fasting since this trigger the releasing o gastric acids in your stomach, which then makes you hungry.

Engage in some other activities, but if you wish to fill your water, drink herbal tea or other drinks free from calories. You may note increased food intake in the non-eating days where you are not limited to any calorie intakes. Intermittent fasting triggers binge food consumption. There could also be cases of cravings, especially after increased levels of cortisol hormone.

Dehydration: Lack of eating may make you forget to take water. You might fail to take note of the thirst cues when fasting.

Fatigue: Intermittent fasting makes you feel tired, especially if you are trying it for the first time. Your body tends to run short of energy and disrupts your sleep patterns, and this comes along with a feeling of being tired.

Irritability: Since intermittent fasting helps in mood regulation, it can as well regulate your appetite. It leads to being depressed and upset.

Intermittent fasting long-term consequences are not known: Since no one knows whether after losing weight, you will maintain the same for some years, studies claim that no relevant evidence to support the extent of intermittent fasting. You are, therefore, always advised to talk to your doctor for sound advice on how you should practice intermittent fasting.

There are precautions that you should undertake when practicing intermittent fasting. Fasting has been there since time immemorial, and in some religions, it is considered as a holy practice. Whatever way, you may start practicing intermittent fasting; you should follow its essential tips to avoid any inconveniences. Therefore, you should:

Ensure that your body is fit for fasting. It is by making sure that you are not pregnant, not under any medication, no health complications, not underage, or even diabetic. If you cannot fast, then you can always change to cleaner eating habits such as eating natural foods and eliminate any sugar, rich, or fatty foods from your diet.

Before starting intermittent fasting, you should always try and consult your doctor. Your doctor will give updates about your health concerns and advise whether the step is necessary or not.

Try and make intermittent fasting fit into your lifestyle. You should never fast during the times you are stressed or under excess exertion. It is advisable if you are a newbie in intermittent fasting to try the 5:2 way of fasting whereby you can fast on the first day of the week, then on Thursdays so that you can prepare to take your favorite meals over the weekend.

Before you start intermittent fasting, do not gorge yourself with a 'last supper,' but you should instead take healthy meals, lean proteins, and vegetables. Fruits have natural sugar and including them in your meal could mean a lot. A little amount of starch could make the meal complete, as well. A meal that has all these nutrients will make your body survive the fasting period.

Prepare your household, body, and thoughts before starting intermittent fasting. It means that you should have enough rest and get prepared emotionally. Think about your aim and how to achieve it. Make sure that you hide or keep out of reach any foods that could tempt you during your fasting period.

Stop pretending to be a hero, even when your body is weak. Do not push your body too hard in the name of fasting. There are some of the symptoms that should be of great concern during your fasting time. You should take note of heart shudders, light-headedness, and general feebleness. It requires the use of common sense because you cannot force your body to do what it cannot.

Do not engage in tough exercises; do light ones. Engage in massages as they help have even blood flow in the body parts full of calories, thus reducing cortisol. Do not burn the muscles for energy while fasting.

Always take your vitamins depending on the method of fasting you choose. That acts as a supplement, especially if in liquid form, as it eases the process of digestion. They help compensate the vitamins lost while fasting.

Never forget to take a lot of water every fasting day. Your urine should alert you if it is not light in color. If not so, drink desirable amounts of water for proper hydration.

Since you are fasting, it is an obstacle to associating with your friends who are having fun, eating chocolates, and drinking wine since you will get tempted to take some. You can indulge in other ways of having fun with your friends. You can pay a visit to the nearest mall, window-shop new clothes or electronics. Avoid grocery stores and any dinner dates. Clear any mouth-watering photos from your gallery.

Avoid getting stressed since stress increases the levels of cortisol, which is responsible for fat storage and muscle breakdown. You can practice yoga, meditating, or having deep breaths. Your body needs enough energy to last you during the fasting period, and so these exercises should be light and not vigorous.

To avoid freaking out, you can always invite your friends to accompany you in doing intermittent fasting. The idea of creating your fasting thread or checking online for any other people doing intermittent fasting can help you master your progress. That is the time that you should focus on mentally cleaning your closet and reflecting on what you are doing.

Avoid 'Victory Binging.' Many people indulge themselves after the fasting period. You should take in a healthy meal and avoid foods that cannot get digested easily. You should take in foods rich in fiber, and if you are alcoholic, remember to take care when resuming.

Chapter 3: The 16/8 Method of Intermittent Fasting

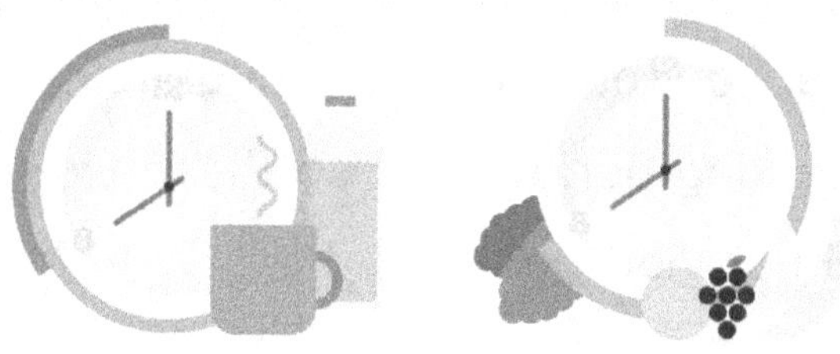

16/8 is a method of fasting done to achieve good health or even lose weight. You have to spend sixteen hours without taking any food, surviving on sugarless drinks such as herbal tea or mineral water. The other eight hours are left open and free for you to eat any meal of your choice. Within these eight hours, you are unrestricted to any specific foods. Intermittent fasting dates back to the time of our ancestors, who could hunt or gather during the day, eat, sleep, and do their fasting during the night. It is all equal to the 16/8 method of intermittent fasting. There are no regulations on which meals you should skip, but the scientists have ascertained that skipping breakfast is okay as no facts that show that breakfast makes you more or less healthier.

Once you have consulted your physician and they recommend the 16/8 for you or tell you that you are fit for this kind of fasting, then you are good to go. It would be an added advantage practicing the 16/8 method if you have tried fasting before, but if you are doing it for the first time, then you need to do it gradually. You can gradually increase your fasting hours from the 5/2 to 12-hour diet plan, then add a little more hours up to 16 hours, then you are good to go. But then again, you should always listen to your body's response to these types of fasting and note the changes.

If you have tried fasting before, your body must have adjusted to energy changes and steaming this method of intermittent fasting with light exercises, and sugarless drinks, keep your body fit. It should not be a point of concern if you find it hard to exercise during fasting periods; it is all normal and okay since human beings' bodies are not the same. It is a method since, after fasting, it gives you enough freedom to consume what you feel like eating, but it should not be an excuse to overeat junk foods. It is strictly clean and healthy meals.

You should avoid highly processed foods during non-fasting times. The following is an example, if not a hint of what you should try eating during the eight-hour non-fasting period:

Early consumption space

8 a.m. – you can take eggs and vegetable scrambles.

Noon – you take apples and almond butter.

Evening – you take chicken and vegetable stir.

If it is midday consumption space, start your day by taking a cup of black tea in the morning.

At 11 a.m., you may banana smoothies.

At 2 p.m. – take avocado toasted bread.

At 4 p.m. – take dark chocolate.

At 6 p.m. – take chicken meatballs with tomato sauce.

If you opt for a late consumption window, drink a cup of black coffee before noon.

At 1 p.m. – take blackberry chia dessert.

At 4 p.m. – take carrots and guacamole.

Then at 9 p.m. – take grilled salmon with veggies.

You can make your meals appear simple but at the same time very healthy. You do not have to restrict yourself to taking five hundred calories, but provided you eat healthy and clean meals within the non-fasting eight hours, you will still achieve your goals. With this method of fasting, you will not be like you would do if you opted for the 5/2 diet plan. The 16/8 is getting popular, even the world's famous personalities and celebrities are practicing this type of intermittent fasting.

Chapter 4: Chronic Degenerative Diseases and Unhealthy Living

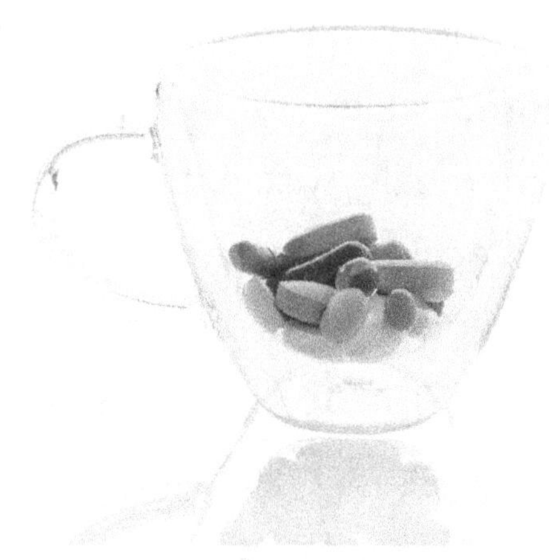

What if diseases were due to nutritional deficiencies and exposure to toxins? This is precisely what constitutes all chronic disease states, and I will cover this subject matter in more in-depth details in the following.

By the end of this book, I want you to become your own authoritative figure and make your own informed decisions. Be skeptical always and think critically, especially when watching mainstream media.

This chapter will be dedicated to chronic degenerative disease states and its correlation to a sedentary lifestyle or unhealthy living. I figured I might as well dedicate a whole chapter to this subject matter, so you can grasp the entire picture of health and wellness and have a multifaceted understanding and not a one-dimensional concept.

The first thing we need to understand is that everything occurs at the level of a cell. What is a cell? A cell is what composes our organs, tissues, bones, and many other bodily appendages. There are many intricate components to a cell, or you can think of them as sub-departments that have their own independent functions. I won't go into details in regard to cell organelles as this is not a science textbook, but I just want you to grasp the fundamental concept of a cell.

In today's modern world, we are bombarded with new prescription drugs almost every other month. Essentially poisons that manipulate our body's biochemistry to suppress inflammation, inhibit the activity or forcefully produce results artificially. The average person doesn't realize that when your interfacing with pharmaceutical drugs to treat chronic diseases, we are playing with fire!

Now I am not saying we don't ever need drugs. I'm not being overly optimistic; however, there is a time and a place for medical intervention through drugs. But, has your doctor ever recommended taking nutrition or even fasting as a viable option to restore your health? Probably not because he doesn't get paid to endorse these kinds of solutions by drug manufacturers, and doctors treat things at the level of symptomologies as oppose to targeting the underlying root problems holistically.

This is what has become of our western medical model, prescription drugs, and invasive procedures that are more or less a band-aid style approach to treating sickness. How is it that our society becomes sicker and sicker with these current standards of treatments? -The answer is simple. These treatments do not work long term but alleviate short term symptoms by ignoring the underlying root casual level.

Every bodily breakdown happens at the level of a cell. Nutrition plays a crucial role in the integrity of our health and wellness. Basically, all chronic degenerative disease states 1. Occur at the level of a cell. 2. Diseases are the lack of nutritional deficiencies and exposure to toxins. Perhaps the premature death of many people here in the industrialized world boils down to the starvation of essential nutrients?

You see, as I mentioned before, prescription drugs have a time and place for usage, and if we are using them to alleviate discomfort in the short term, I'm completely fine with that and even recommend it. However, when doctors start prescribing patient's prescription drugs long term as viable options for treatment, then I put my foot down and cannot stand for this. Prescription drugs are one of the leading causes of death in America, and your doctor is certainly not helping the cause! You see, all you do is mask symptoms with drugs without ever tackling the root problem.

Drugs only poison the body to cover symptoms and essentially creating a falsehood of "good health," and we think this is ok?

So okay, by now, you understand the determinantal effects of prescription drugs, but can nutrition and fasting really be used as medicine to treat chronic diseases? Yes! Absolutely, we see this time and time again, people reversing their diseases with the right nutritional protocol and elimination of food toxicity.

I mentioned earlier in the last chapter how the body is an amazing piece of sophisticated machinery that only requires the right raw materials to function optimally.

Still, don't believe me that everyone has an intelligent self-healing system that is inherent within our body? The next time you cut your finger, observe and see what happens, and you will see the marvelous intelligence and self-repair mechanism of your body at work. What happens when you cut yourself? You bleed yes, but what happens after without you even thinking of giving a command?

Your body starts to repair itself on its own! You didn't even need to think it! Platelets come to the cover and patch up the wound in a matter of seconds, and the healing process begins almost instantly. Now, do you see how your body is a healing system capable of taking care of itself as long as the right conditions are met?

Now let us discuss nutrition. You need to understand the fundamentals of nutrition in order to use it correctly. The following are the fundamentals of nutrition.

Fundamental Nutritional Building Blocks

- Protein – best sources whey powder, bone soup & eggs.

- Fats – Essential fatty acids, salmon, Herring, Sardines, Halibut.

- Carbs – Leafy green vegetables, cabbage, Romanian salad, carrots, cucumbers, and you can also add olive or coconut oils as dressing.

- Water - Filtered Water. Our bodies are electrical systems and use electrical currents when minerals and water are combined in conjunction.

- Two Types of Vitamins: Fat-soluble and Water-soluble.

Fat-soluble = Vitamin D, A, E, K.

Water soluble = B Vitamin complex and Vitamin C.

- Minerals – Zinc, Silica, copper, magnesium, chromium, and vanadium.

- Trace minerals & nutrients – selenium, NAC.

- Probiotics – Lactobacillus acidophilus, Bifidobacterium bifidum.

All the above-listed nutrition constitutes your fundamental building blocks for health and wellness.

Inflammation

We all have had some sort of inflammation at some point or the other in our life. We take the medication in order to alleviate inflammation and the inconvenience it brings to us, and although relieving symptoms that irritate us in the short term is ok for comfort, however its when we do this in the long term without addressing the root problem.

So, what is inflammation? First of all, we need to understand why inflammation occurs in the first place! Inflammation is apart of our immune system and is our body's defensive response to something that triggers our system. That's right inflammation is our body's way of protecting itself from an intruder, thus instead of knocking down the immune system as the solution, we need to figure out what is causing the immune system to be triggered.

That would be the most logical move according to deductive reasoning; thus, we need to find out why our body is responding in a defensive fashion and what exactly is the catalyst to this trigger. Therefore, anytime you have inflammation, you need to think about what is causing this to happen? Long term use of immune system suppression through drugs can literally shut down your immune response for other essential things. For instance, imagine you're a long-term user of a prescription drug that suppresses inflammation causing pain for arthritis, and you get into a car accident, or you have a nasty slip and fall. Your recovery from the accident will be almost non-existent, and you could potentially die easier because your immune system has been suppressed for so long.

Do you see the dangers of long-term use of immune-suppressing drugs? And I should say any prescription drug for that matter. There are really only three ways your immune system can be activated, and that's through your respiratory tract, digestive tract, and skin contact. In other words, breathing, eating, and direct skin contact is really the only possible entry points where your body mounts a defensive response which means inflammation!

For most people, it is usually eating! Thus, any sort of immune response associated with food allergies should give you an indication of what is triggering your immune response. You need to figure out which foods are causing your flare-up.

All Chronic Diseases Starts at the Level of a Cell

In today's modern world, we find ourselves assaulted on so many fronts at different levels from synthetic food, addiction, and habitual forming substances, chemical additives, and much more.

The first thing we need to understand is that the body degenerates at the level of a cell, and the various disease states we see manifestations of today are simply degeneration occurring at different parts of the body. In essence, your body is falling apart at different structural levels, and we classify these as different categories of diseases depending on what department of the body the chronic degeneration occurs at.

We are misled to focus on specific components of the body when we fall ill, instead of treating ourselves holistically. After all our bodies work in harmony at the most cellular level, systems and cells communicate with each other, signaling, up-regulating, etc.

The human body is composed of cells, and all diseases fundamentally start off at the cellular level before spreading to the different systems of the body. Humans are composed of a trillion and trillions of cells.

From a simplistic standpoint, the body can be broken down into two things, cells and the extracellular matrix. Thus, in order to understand the degenerative disease process, we need to understand things at the level of a cell and the matrix.

These cells we are composed of are nothing short of a miracle and contain organelles structures, which are sub-compartments of operating machinery that have various functions. The outside of the cell, known as the membrane, works like an information chip processor, and inside at the epicenter, we find the blueprint known as DNA. Our cells perform incredible tasks, precision action, producing various chemicals at a methodical choreography.

I am just trying to describe to you how elaborate, complex, intricate, and beautifully crafted every single human being is. The point I am trying to drive across is we are designed divinely, and our bodies possess the necessary tools to function but only need the correct raw materials. Input the wrong materials (junk foods), and you will pay dearly with the consequences of poor health.

Good health is our birthright, and no doctor, surgeon, pharmacist, and any other health care professional has any right over your divinely bestowed gift and birthright as a human being. We don't need to depend on this "medical model" for good health or any other authoritative figure because the truth has been right under our noses this whole time, and that is we are in control!

Now I am not saying the innovations and advancements in technology, especially in regard to medicine, are all wasted. No, I am not saying that at all; however, there is a time and a place for medical intervention. But when dealing with chronic diseases that are onset by lifestyle choices that we control, then no doctor has any business with our health by manipulating our biochemistry with drugs and literally butchering our human appendages.

We must understand that all chronic diseases are a by-product of cell starvation (lack of nutrients), toxification (sugar and pollutants), and suffocation (lack of oxygen). So, it doesn't matter what you are struggling with, whether it's the heart, bone, nerves, muscle, pancreas, etc. all disease initially occurs at the level of the cell.

The issue with modern medicine is we focus too much on the specifics without considering the entire context. There is nothing wrong with being specific as we need to be in order to be precise; however, we must not neglect the context of the situation and grasp everything holistically.

Now let us talk a little about the cellular matrix that also makes up the human body. The matrix is where all the electrical energy and bio-chemical synthesis occurs that drives all the incredible work of the cells found in our body. Thus, you can think of the matrix as the support of the cells that provide or feeds the cells with hormones, nutrients, oxygen, and anything else you can think of. Also, the matrix is responsible for draining all the poisons, and by-products cells produce.

So now you understand the concept of cells and the matrix, so now I would like to now talk about how the onset of the disease process begins. The first point of break down for almost any chronic degenerative disease is at the point of your digestive system! The digestive system becomes compromised and dysfunctional, thus causing a wide array of physiological distress. It is really a cascading effect that systemically affects your entire body.

So, after your digestive system breaks down, your blood sugar system goes awry and then your adrenal thyroid complex dysfunctions. The point I want to emphasize here is if you focus on correcting these three components of health, digestive system, blood sugar system, and the adrenal thyroid complex, everything else will fall into place! Simple right?

You're probably thinking right now, but what about if you have arthritis or any other chronic disease that is not directly connected to those three systems? There seems to be a disconnect, but you need to understand that these three systems are behind all other bodily structures, so wouldn't it make sense to strengthen these systems first in order to have a "domino effect" of good health?

So now you understand the concept of cells and the matrix, so now I would like to now talk about how the onset of the disease process begins. The first point of break down for almost any chronic degenerative disease is at the point of your digestive system! The digestive system becomes compromised and dysfunctional, thus causing a wide array of physiological distress. -It is really a cascading effect that systemically affects your entire body.

So, after your digestive system breaks down, your blood sugar system goes awry and then your adrenal thyroid complex dysfunctions. The point I want to emphasize here is if you focus on correcting these three components of health, digestive system, blood sugar system, and the adrenal thyroid complex, everything else will fall into place! Simple right?

You're probably thinking right now, but what about if you have arthritis or any other chronic disease that is not directly connected to those three systems? There seems to be a disconnect, but you need to understand that these three systems are behind all other bodily structures, so wouldn't it make sense to strengthen these systems first in order to have a "domino effect" of good health?

Imagine your growing an apple tree, but for this tree to bear ripe, healthy fruits, you need to first put your focus on the ground or soil it is being planted into. You need to build the foundation right to get the desired result and, in this case, is the fruit. In this same manner, the three systems interconnected to the entire body need to be functioning optimally for pristine health.

Hence, all the chronic disease states we are plagued with induced by our poor lifestyle choices can be thought to be the "leaves" being produced at the core of the entire breakdown process of these three systems. Now, this is a profound realization because all we need to do is take corrective measures and focus on the root problem of diseases.

So, to recap all this your living the typical American sedentary lifestyle, consume junk foods daily which lack nutrients, possess toxins (sugar), and poor oxygenation from our industrialized society, and in conjunction with lack of exercise leads to obesity and is the jumping-off point of many other chronic degenerative disease states.

Healing Strategies

- Nutrition
- Oxygenation (Deep breathing)
- Rest
- Exercise
- Intermittent Fasting
- Eliminating food toxicity

Health is so simple, don't complicate things. The body needs proper nutrition, fresh oxygen, and small amounts of stress to stimulate growth via exercise, periods of rest, cleanses through fasting, and of course, eliminating food poison from our diet.

Acne Case Study – Closing Thoughts

In a remote island called Kitava located near the province of Papua New Guinea, we find native inhabitants with a population density of 10,000–12,000 people. Untouched by western influence in regard to the food supply, we find these people consuming diets rich in essential fats, vitamins, and minerals.

We found no prevalence of chronic ailments of the western hemisphere, and it appears that these people don't seem to struggle with our type of degenerative disease states such as diabetes, dementia, high blood pressure, heart disease, etc. How can this be? Would you write this off as "it is in their genetics" to have good health? Obviously, not that is silly as genetics play a secondary role in the outcome of your health, and the primary influence on genetics is lifestyle choices.

Let's take a closer look at the case study conducted by professor Steffan Lindeberg who is a certified doctor (GP) and is a huge proponent of evolutionary nutrition. Over the course of 800+ days, no signs of acne were reported in any of the population! Acne is such a common problem here in the western world and can be considered a disease of the industrialized world.

Absolutely none of the population suffered from a chronic skin disease known as acne that plagues the western world. And there was no magic fruit or pill that they took, which gave them clear skin and good health. However, their diets consisted of fish, coconuts, some fruits, yams, and other vegetables. In other words, the people of Kitava consumed "wholefoods," and these foods were not processed or altered by chemicals but are completely natural. Their diets have not changed since the time of their native first-generation ancestors.

They had generations upon generations of smooth and clear skin and no reports of other chronic disease states either simply because of their lifestyle choices. The interesting thing is when the western diet was introduced to the populace, then the only acne started to emerge and surface! Again, we see the correlation between chronic diseases and the standard American western diet. Wholefoods vs. refined foods, and at this point, it is indisputable even to conceive you can't use wholefoods or even fast as medicine. Simply changing your diet to a wholefood primarily plant-based one can prevent chronic degenerative diseases.

Chapter 5: Times When Women Should Avoid Intermittent Fasting

As a woman, you should note that intermittent fasting has become one of the favorite ways of losing weight or even improving your general health. Starvation has been reported to be a fair practice as it positively changes many people's lives. If you have been fasting, you must have heard a notion that fasting is not healthy for women, despite the many positive impacts it has on their bodies. Intermittent fasting has different impacts on men and women. It is less beneficial to women as compared to men.

There exist myths that many women experience changes in their menstrual periods after starting intermittent fasting. These changes may take place since women's bodies are reactive, especially after the restriction of calories. When you take fewer calories, the hypothalamus part of the brain is always affected. This means that women should try intermittent fasting with shorter periods. The affected hormones tend to interfere with the ovaries, and that is why the menstrual periods are affected. This brings out the concern of when to avoid intermittent fasting as a woman.

Intermittent Fasting and Menstruation

As recurrent fasting grows into a supplementary general, women who starve on a regular basis might have queries about how starving could impact their multiplicative sequence, hormones, and multiplicative well-being. Even though there is some degree of investigation on how recurrent fasting or ketogenic foods may influence multiplicative sequences in persons, you can take some hints from the study, including further metabolic and way of life characters and performances such as heaviness, workout and caloric constraint.

Whether it is not well-thought-out well-meaning of study or it is well-thought-out "ancient updates," there are shortages of scientific studies on the way ketogenic nutrition and sporadic starving might influence female's multiplicative sequences together with multiplicative fitness. On the other hand, you are aware that caloric consumption, exercises, and heaviness might affect the procreative hormone sequence. For instance, life-threatening procedures of caloric limitation, mass loss, workout, and dietary deficits can all lead to "amenorrhea," unbalanced otherwise bounced menstrual periods.

Calories constraint, for instance, can be said to be a "stressor" handled in your mind and might as well adjust discharge of gender hormone via an axis known as the "Hypothalamic-Pituitary-Gonadal (HPG)" alignment. Giving birth, as well as productiveness, is controlled by the hormone of the HPG alignment.

Women who are not acquiring enough caloric intakes to support HPG axis could possibly experience irregular menses; this is with regard to intermittent fasting. Shortened, this insinuates that on condition that a lady lacks sufficient nutritious or breakdown vigor to sustain her during the prenatal period, your (her) body will send signals to your mind to shut down the multiplicative sequence. Due to this purpose, females attempting to get expectant might be cautious of starving for lengthier than twenty-four hours at a period or evocatively limiting their calorie consumption by fasting, particularly if they are by now at a strong heaviness. It is improbable that an uncommon time of starving to every month will fling away your monthly periods' sequence, even though considerable caloric constraint might.

Undesirable energy stability or caloric limitation in the undeveloped women may as well have the consequences of adjourning adolescence through impacts on the HPG alignment and neuro-hormones. Absent or irregular menstrual periods are caused by excessive exercise; this is an important piece of information for women. Currently, if you are not thinking about having a baby or getting pregnant at this position in your life, then you should know that your body is. The procreative system within a woman is designed to support the prenatal period right from the time you experience your period until such a period that you stop menstruating, that is menopause. In order to support and maintain a healthy pregnancy, females ought to have certain amounts of energy as well as nutrients, acquired from food and then kept as fats, to be able to support their wellbeing pregnancy. Women's bodies have the capability to distinguish the times these energy stores are down and are able to, in essence 'switch' your procreative sequences so that you do not get pregnant. The means through which this takes place is, in fact, quite intricate and needs a weak sense of balance of signals to be communicated amid the brain, the pituitary glands as well as the ovaries. Characteristically, the time a woman regains heaviness and (or) returns back to a diet rich in nutrients, and the usual menstrual sequences will come back.

Various outside and interior contributions of the mind are key rulers of the multiplicative fitness and menstrual sequences.

These contributions can comprise aspects such as your liveliness condition, your dietary and calories consumption plus spending, constant worry points, and also exterior contributions into the heartbeat. Those numerous contributions work via the HPG alignment by influencing the work of "the gonadotropin-releasing hormone (GnRH)." This hormone's role is to be accountable for the discharge of "the follicle-stimulating hormone (FSH) "plus" the luteinizing hormone (LH) "to the bloodstream from the pituitary gland in the frontal part found in the brain of a human being. Follicle-stimulating Hormone, in addition, the Luteinizing Hormone, as soon as they are released, move to a woman's ovaries to help the discharge of follicles of the ovary, which comprise of the egg cells, the creation of estrogen plus progesterone as well as testosterone. Gonadotropin-releasing Hormone is seen as a neuro-hormone; therefore, it is secreted from exceptional gonadotropin-releasing hormone neurons found in the brain, precisely the hypothalamus.

Your reproductive health and menstrual cycle can be influenced by external factors such as stress, or your expressive and interactive state. Circadian light-dark is similarly another external factor that affects our reproductive health, and we don't often think. Even though a number of women reside in regions that they get approximately twelve days, twelve nights, people tend to have more irregular menstrual cycles when they go through tremendously extended days or tremendously extended nights, such as women living in the poles.

For example, the Hypothalamic-Pituitary-Gonadal alignment is competent to adapt and is similarly adjusted by stress hormone communicating with the inclusion corticosterone, from the hypothalamic-pituitary-adrenal (HPA), and this is because procreation and continued existence require to be synchronized and reasonable. Constant worry, together with constant psychological worry, can unhelpfully influence reproduction in a large number of the mammalian kind, not excluding the humans. Due to nervous tension, women are able to experience ovarian cycle disruption, as well as upstream gonadotropin synthesis and secretion.

The physical pressure and the long-lasting pints of cortisol hormone (a type of stress hormone that disrupts the multiplicative sequence) can be decreased concentrated by healthy points of reasonable workout, slumber, and mindfulness. Fasting is complex, especially when it is based on the stress points—fasting is over and over again well-thought-out to be an enclosed or "good" worry, like workout, but you can ask yourself, how much can a woman fast without getting her periods affected?

There are no widespread principles or guidelines on how many times one should starve per month, this is because of its problematic nature and relevance of its application, for example, it would be harmless to a woman struggling to come to be pregnant or to stop any menstrual sequence variations. For any woman, there exists a lot of personal unpredictability in menstrual sequences. Despite the fact that reasonable time-limited feeding (about 12-14 hours for each diurnal or fewer) or else in frequent fasting days underneath twenty-four hours are almost certainly harmless, diet excellence, calories consumption and Body Mass Index are expected to regulate the influences of irregular starvation and keto regimes on procreative wellbeing.

When nutrient deficits and prolonged hypoglycemia or low blood sugar is caused by your intermittent fasting practice, it is possible that the hypothalamic, the pituitary and the gonadal axis will be impacted, and interrupt the secretion of the procreative hormones. At hand are some studies in animal reproductions (undeveloped rats) that have advanced the idea that nutritional restriction through alternating fasting might damagingly impact hypothalamus-hypophyseal-gonadal alignment and then in a similar measure the reproduction. In one of the studies, rats that were starved on a daily basis (one week of human starvation is similar to a day of starving a rat) which results in up to a forty percent reduction in caloric consumption, went through significant fluctuations in their body mass, estrous cycle, blood sugar, as well as serum estradiol, testosterone, LH levels and GnRH appearance.

How then can the Ramadan period on fasting influence menstrual sequences?

As it is described above, some of the factors that have been established to influence menstrual sequences comprise severe workout, weight loss, and psychological stressors. But then again, some research inquiries have found that irregular eating forms, unusually minute concentrations of leptin (connected to liveliness deficiency), and Ramadan observation as some of the subjects that can influence menstruation. In fact, Ramadan fasting including other procedures of irregular fasting is as well dangerous for expectant women, since researchers have exposed alterations in procreative hormones and reduced weight addition in women who starve for the duration of the Ramadan month.

A study in 2013, a study of eighty female undergraduates from "Hamedan University of Medical Sciences" established that persons who starved for additional fifteen times for the period of Ramadan month remained more probable to have menstrual irregularities, together with uncommon or missed menstrual periods, abnormal flow of blood or weighty or lengthy menstruation. These results continued for three months, succeeding Ramadan period. Most of the partakers were standard heaviness or slender.

On the other hand, a different study on females with Polycystic Ovary Syndrome (POS) revealed that

Ramadan observance through food abstinence could have accommodating moments on the points of anxiety hormone such as cortisol, whereby with restricted impacts on procreative hormone like the "follicle-stimulating hormone" and "luteinizing hormone." These high points the necessity for additional study on the way starvation might affect women in different ways. For instance, weighty or obese women suffering from stimulating matters may position themselves to the benefit of irregular fasting through time-restricted eating, even if it comprises of a sub-optimal eating plan (for instance, evening eating) just like that of Ramadan starving.

During the period of Ramadan, Muslim devotees are faced with an observance that requires the refrain from eating from morning to evening for all periods. Such a form of eating pattern may stimulate procreative hormone sequences both unwaveringly but also meanderingly through interference with a heartbeat and sleeping preparations, particularly since refraining from nutrition and drink throughout the day outlines that back up strong circadian paces. It is clearly recognized that menstrual sequences influence the circadian clock and sleep through gender hormones such as estrogen. For instance, daytime paces of melatonin and cortisol hormones transform during the course of the menstrual round. On the backside, disruption of menstrual progression is correlated with the circadian paces. For instance, women who toilet hours during night time are more expected to have menstrual irregularities and extended sequences.

Both the change of working environment and irregular estrogen gesturing can also impact the appearance of the 24-hourly *CLOCK* genetic factor, with downstream insinuations for procreative fitness and also the growth and progression of breast cancer cells. Day by day measures in the multiplication of cells safeguard your body from ardent cancer cells. Quotidian interference aids cancer cells multiply by allowing them to divide "round the clock."

The disruption and alterations of existing biological patterns, as it usually happens in shift jobs, jet lags, sleep deficiency, have significant linkage with the disruption of the reproductive function. Such alteration or modification includes reduced conception rates, distorted hormonal discharge rhythms, increased miscarriage numbers, and greater than before the danger of breast cancer. Disconcerted hormonal patterns control the appearance of rhythms of the clock genes as a result of the susceptible nature of female health through the desynchronizing of work schedules.

Clock gene expression in the uterus is modified by the clock gene expression and "the suprachiasmatic nucleus" found in the brain, the location of the most important "circadian clock mechanism. "

There is still a lot at hand that limits the knowledge and recognition of how precisely the 24-hour pace interference impacts menstruation and procreative well-being, even though there is a huge possibility it has to do with alterations in hormone discharge. The ovary gives the impression of having its personal day to day clock; as soon as this clock is available and tuned with diurnal rhythms somewhere else in your body, multiplicative sequence can rise. But then again what does recurrent fasting have to do with this situation? Intermittent fasting predominantly time-limited eating, may facilitate you uphold healthy circadian measures by nutrient indications, in the condition that nutrient consumption within the standard points of activities (for example, in the course of the day) is upheld.

Alternatively, being otherwise healthy, you may not wish to starve in the course of the twelve hours and consume simply later in the sunset, since this might lead to interrupted circadian pulses that may affect the hormone intensities. Denoting that it may, for the time being, raise the stress levels as well as cortisol but at the end of the day have a constructive, anti-inflammatory outcome if practiced on a regular basis.

What do you know about by what method ketogenic diet or other nutrition may influence your menstrual period and procreative wellbeing?

Scientists are yet on the verge of identifying and successfully defining whether ketogenetic dietary consumption is advantageous in clinical settings–you might have a minute idea or less information if any, the influence of these foods on women's multiplicative sequences. On the other hand, you also know that gaining weight (being obese) has a destructive impact on reproductive fitness and success rates in attaining expectancy. From the viewpoint, a keto dietary consumption like a heaviness-loss involvement before the prenatal period is probable to help the procreative wellbeing of weighty and overweight persons.

There is no hesitation that the overall health of a human being is impacted by their weight, so it should not come as a surprise that reproductive health is affected too. Women who are overweight or underweight might have unbalanced menstrual periods or fight with unproductiveness.

Fascinatingly, there are studies that have explored the way the ketogenic foods might advance the multiplicative well-being of females with PCOS. However, additional inquiries are required to identify how keto meals influence females with no PCOS. Like an all-purpose rule, when are encouraged to converse with their physicians before they begin a new diet, but especially caution is to women are heavy with a child, or attempting to be pregnant; this is because correct nutrition is an indispensable factor in supporting and maintain a strong pregnancy.

The existing substantiation lays no doubt on the reduction of circulating insulin levels as a result of plummeting carbohydrate load, recover the hormonal difference, and lead to a recommencement of ovulation to advance the rates of pregnancy. The conclusions of the assessment established that minimal carbohydrate foods with less than forty-five percent carbohydrates, optimizes productiveness as recorded in some scientific categories, predominantly for heavy and overweight females having PCOS.

Can nutrition lead to additional cramping in the course of periods or weightier flows?

A quick search on the internet about cramps and diet will lead you to numerous various pieces of information, signifying that a variety of diets, meals, or enhancements all can lead to or relieve menstrual cramping. Preliminary investigation in a credible peer-reviewed journal discovers that less-fat veggie foods and three to four servings of dairy food each day might be useful in decreasing menstruation cramping.

A less-fat veggie food was positively linked to an enlarged serum gender-hormone fastening, globulin absorption, together with dysmenorrheal [painful periods] duration, reductions in body heaviness, and strength, as well as premenstrual warning sign length. The dietary influences on estrogen activity mediate the symptoms inherent in cramping.

Monitor It

So that you can be a hale and hearty female irregular faster, just be conscious plus observe your procreative sequence. More or less the existing use of LIFE starving monitoring app, consumers' preferred procreative fitness and menstruation monitoring apps which consists of "Clue" (menstruation tracker), "Glow" (a productiveness calculator), "Natural Cycles" (used to monitor the cycle), plus" the Ava sequence" are important for your daily updates. In the vent that anything is different from your usual pattern, it is appropriate and advisable to contact your physician.

Watching intrusions to your menstrual periods is an approachable method of defining and identifying whether you are required to decrease the number of times or periods that you are refraining from eating for every month, mainly on the condition that you are attempting or preparing to be expectant. The uncluttered query is the way abstinence from food may influence the efficiency of the natal controlling dose–you need to obtain more information about this from gynecologist having that there are limited on this topic.

Chapter 6: Why Wholefoods Are Essential

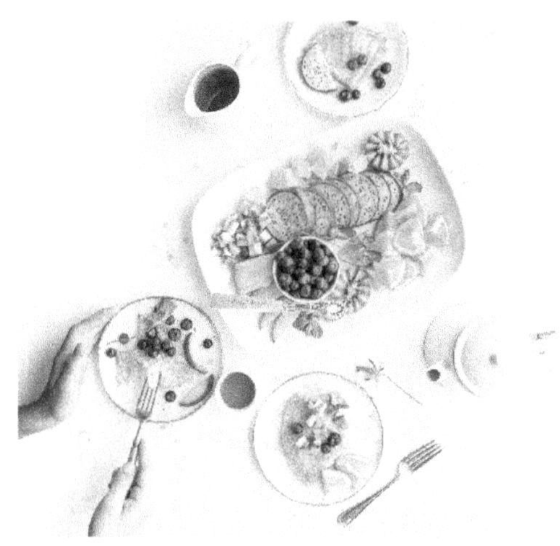

In this chapter, I will discuss the importance of wholefoods, why they're beneficial to us, and 30 recommended wholefoods and delicious recipes you can try yourself.

But before I do that, I wanted to ask a question, have you noticed that most major supermarkets carry almost no "wholefoods"? Most of their shelves are stocked with refined foods that can be found inside a cardboard box with mostly empty calories. This is because refined foods have longer shelf lives and last for extended periods of time because they have removed all the raw, whole, and fresh, natural ingredients.

The thing about whole foods is that although they are a powerhouse for essential vitamins and minerals; however, since they are fresh foods, they don't last as long as refined foods. Now from a business standpoint of view and perspective, wholefoods would be a liability because you can't make as much money with foods that perish and don't last as long.

This is partly the reason why food manufacturers develop refined foods with preservatives and other additives to keep food's lifespan extended so they can sell to us the consumer and make more profits.

Wholefoods are the perfect food they contain the perfect balance and are the most nutritionally dense foods we can find on the planet. The issue is due to modern-day agriculture and mineral-depleted soil supply, and we are left with foods that lack proper nutrition. That's not to say whole foods cannot produce. They certainly can be; however, the majority of farmers have to use additives to maintain its value.

As you know, there are many minerals and vitamins that wholefoods contain. The chief among them is vitamin C, which is essential to our very existence. Vitamin C is used for a myriad of biochemical functions, and best of all, you cannot overdose on it because it is water-soluble. Animals in the wild make their own vitamin C! – Humans, guerrillas, and guinea pigs are the only known species who cannot produce their own vitamin C within their bodies.

The early European settlers upon arriving in North America were plagued with a disease known as scurvy. This was a nasty disease that literally made you fall apart, classical hallmark signs of scurvy are gingivitis, anemia, sore joints, and degeneration of collagen. Native aboriginals of the land introduced a remedy which was by boiling the leaves and bark of trees into an elixir and served it to the European settlers who suffered from scurvy.

Guess what? They were cured! Their disease started to reverse as soon as they drank the concoction, and surprise, surprise the reason this happened

is because the leaves and tree barks that were boiled into drinks contained vitamin C! (ascorbic acid) Again, history has shown us how using nutrition as medicine is a viable treatment option to chronic diseases, and case in point that most degenerative diseases at the core are actually nutritional deficiencies! Not random or solely "genetic" causes.

Therefore, let this be a lesson to us here in the 21st century and take this experience from the early European settlers and apply it to our lives. What if chronic diseases at the core were the result of nutritional deficiencies that manifested as bodily breakdown. Remember, a chronic disease is a breakdown of the body due to poor lifestyle choices and is different from an external bacterial or viral disease.

So, we know that nutrition can help strengthen the body and reverse chronic diseases, but why do we neglect it in today's modern medicine even though history shows us otherwise? Why do we look to only solve short term symptoms neglecting the root cause? Who's vested interest does it serve to keep the masses perpetually ill?

-Imagine the number of pharmacies and even hospitals that would go out of business if they endorsed wholefoods and an active lifestyle? I will leave it to your imagination to formulate your own answer as I have provided you all the necessary info to help you make an informed decision.

Plant-Based Foods

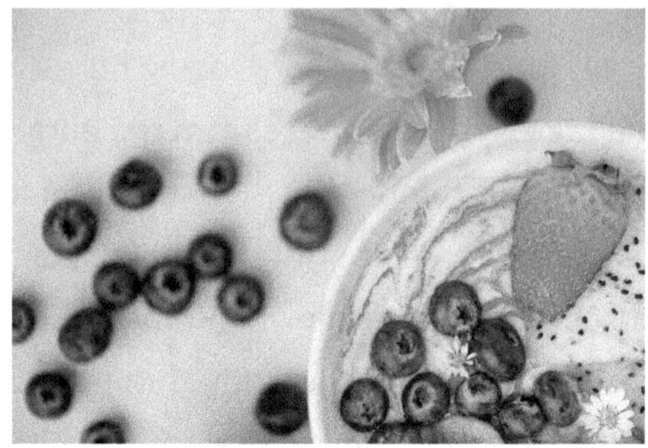

So, what exactly are whole foods? Well, generally speaking, wholefoods are plants based on foods that are raw and minimally processed. Primarily vegetables are where you want to get your main source of wholefoods leafy greens, beets, bell peppers, cucumbers, cabbage, carrots, and you can even add spices or dressing to enhance flavor.

Fruits are also considered whole foods, but you got to be careful with fruits because they do contain sugar, thus eating fruits in minimal amounts alongside vegetables is ok. A lot of advocates of nutrition recommend wholegrain foods, but if you read this far into the book, you can imagine why I do not recommend whole grain foods. The only exception to this rule is brown rice, but again in minimal amounts too.

If we look at animals in the wild, whether guerillas or elephants, we observe extremely powerful creatures, yet they're dieting consists of plant-based foods! – Now I am not endorsing you don't need meat, but the case and point I am trying to establish are such majestic, and powerful creatures in the wild consume whole foods that consist of a plant-based diet.

Do we see these wild animals plagued with chronic diseases like us humans here in the industrialized world? We don't see obese, diabetic, or any other form of chronic disease affecting animals in the wild, yet humans, despite the great strides in our technological advancements and industrial feats, still struggle with common health problems at alarming rates.

Thus, it makes sense when we see these almost miraculous results of disease reversal when patients are put on a plant-based diet. People go off their insulin medication, lowers cholesterol, stabilizes blood sugar levels, blood pressure normalizes, weight loss, and many other chronic symptoms reverse.

The old adage proves to be true "you are what you eat," but more specifically are what you absorb. Now I don't only endorse strictly eating plants although that is a healthy option, I am a firm believer of balance, and you need a good source of protein from lean, unprocessed meats. My top two picks are wild Alaskan Salmon and lean chicken breast.

If we look at animals in the wild, whether guerillas or elephants, we observe extremely powerful creatures, yet they're dieting consists of plant-based foods! Now I am not endorsing you don't need meat, but the case and point I am trying to establish are such majestic, and powerful creatures in the wild consume whole foods that consist of a plant-based diet.

Do we see these wild animals plagued with chronic diseases like us humans here in the industrialized world? We don't see obese, diabetic, or any other form of chronic disease affecting animals in the wild, yet humans, despite the great strides in our technological advancements and industrial feats, still struggle with common health problems at alarming rates.

Thus, it makes sense when we see these almost miraculous results of disease reversal when patients are put on a plant-based diet. People go off their insulin medication, lowers cholesterol, stabilizes blood sugar levels, blood pressure normalizes, weight loss, and many other chronic symptoms reverse.

The old adage proves to be true "you are what you eat," but more specifically are what you absorb. Now I don't only endorse strictly eating plants although that is a healthy option, I am a firm believer of balance, and you need a good source of protein from lean, unprocessed meats. My top two picks are wild Alaskan Salmon and lean chicken breast, preferably organic. I know organic meat can get expensive, but even the lean meat found at grocery stores is a better alternative than processed and red meats, which are responsible for many chronic diseases you find at your local supermarket.

From anti-oxidants, plant phytonutrients, vitamins, essential fats, and minerals, there is no reason why you shouldn't incorporate wholefoods into your diet. The mounting scientific body of evidence cannot be disputed of the enormous health benefits and preventive measures whole foods provide. You reduce the risk of cancer, obesity, diabetes, high blood pressure, and almost any other chronic degenerative disease you can think of.

Support for wholefoods primarily plant-based diets is given by the American Cancer Society, American College of Cardiology, Harvard School of Public Health, and the National Institute of Health. As you can see, I am not the only advocate for wholefoods as a method of prevention from the many chronic diseases that assail us in today's modern world.

What is the Ketogenic Diet?

There is this buzzword being thrown around in the health and fitness industries known as the "ketogenic diet." But what exactly is the ketogenic diet, and how is it beneficial to our health?

The ketogenic diet is a moderate protein diet, low in carbohydrates but high in fat. Consisting of 60-80% fat, 10-20% carbs, and 20-25% protein in your diet. The key here is to create an environment that induces fat burning by having readily available fuel by burning fat present within your body with minimal carbs and moderate protein. This forces your body to switch from sugar burning to fat burning.

You ideally want to become a fat burner because if you were to compare it gram for gram in regard to fuel-burning fat is superior because it's a lot cleaner. Don't believe me? Okay, well, have you ever tried cooking with sugar? When it is heated, it leaves behind a sticky, crusty, caramel, and hard to clean residue. Now imagine this occurring in your body when you use sugar as fuel.

Fat, on the other hand, doesn't leave this kind of residue and burns more efficiently. Our body's sugar burning process creates something called "advanced glycated end products," also known as AGES.

You can consider sugar to be a dirty fuel that leaves residue behind and destruction in its wake. So, what's special about burning fat? Well, for one, when you start utilizing fat for fuel, you produce these molecules called "ketones," and the ongoing process of burning ketones is known as ketosis.

Ketones are high energy compounds and very easy for the body to use from the brain, muscle, heart, and even for the liver. It's so ironic how we have conditioned ourselves through the misinformation that fats in our diets make us fat, and although this can be true for saturated and trans-fats, not in the case of healthy fats. It seems really counterintuitive that eating fat can help us lose weight, but the actual fact is that fat induces "fat-burning" mechanisms within our bodies.

The mainstream media's way of thinking is low fat and high carbs, and this is what they promote you should be eating, but this is fundamentally erroneous on a biological scale and for the purpose of weight loss. Thus, remember the more fat you eat in the presence of low carbs and moderate protein will enable you to switch from sugar burning to fat burning.

Already you can see the multiple benefits of the ketogenic diet, cleaner source of fuel, lose weight, and have more energy to utilize!

Difference Between Paleo and Ketogenic Diet

Also known as the caveman "diet," the Paleo diet is a high protein diet, moderate fat, and low carb regiment. It is similar to the ketogenic diet but has switched the focus on high protein as opposed to high fat. Now both these diets are extremely effective for losing weight, and both these regiments understand the concept of keeping your consumption of carbs low, especially refined carbs.

However, I prefer the ketogenic diet over the paleo diet. Why? Simply because with the paleo diet's focus on high protein, this can potentially cause problems. As you know, protein in large quantities, if not utilized via exercise, also converts into sugar!

Who should go on the ketogenic diet? I recommend anyone and everyone to go onto this diet because of its multiple benefits and, most importantly, how it forces the body to shift its metabolic process from burning sugar to fat burning. I truly believe this is the way humans are designed to eat because the body prefers using ketones and deriving your energy from sugar can cause problematic issues.

The ketogenic diet is arguably one of the best lifestyle changes to make it has anti-cancer, anti-aging, anti-seizure, and many more benefits to it.

So, I've spoken a lot about fat, and it is good for you. But what exactly is the type of fats you need to be eating? When I say fats, I am not referring to the French fries, saturated, trans fat, and hydrogenated fats. When I refer to fats, I am talking about eggs, lard, butter, cheese, fish, yogurt, and organ meats. When selecting fats, you got to ensure they are minimally processed, not cooked, and are whole fats.

Chapter 7: How You Can Identify Your Body Type as a Woman

You see, the fact is that not everybody has the same genetics, and therefore what works for them specifically may not necessarily work for you. We are all unique individuals who possess different physical traits, and to follow a generic work-out routine and expect to get shredded within a week is not realistic.

Thus, in this chapter, I wanted to cover exercise routines and body types to give you a grasp of the entire picture of health and wellness. Although diet is fundamental to weight loss, it works even betters, and its effects are amplified in conjunction with exercise.

I've taken the liberty to give you a specifically designed exercise regimen for your precise body type. All you have to is identify your body type through the criteria I provided and follow the regiment catered towards you.

- **Ectomorph – lean** and lanky, has difficulty building muscle, high metabolism, and has a tendency to remain slender.

- **Endomorph –** Bigger body composition, high body fat, pear shape liked and has a tendency to store fat.
- **Mesomorph –** The more favorable body type. Naturally muscular, and possess responsive muscle cells.

The Ectomorph characterized by long extremities in specific their arms and legs. These individuals tend to have a hard time gaining weight and building muscle and are noted for having slender builds. They don't have to be extremely picky about what they eat since their metabolism burns fat really quickly. But keep this in context. Any poor eating habits can eventually lead to obesity. Work out consists of heavier weights and fewer reps.

Ectomorph Exercises

- Stretch for two minutes

- Barbell Bench Press 4 sets, 4-8 reps, no more than eight reps

- Incline Dumbbell Press 4 sets, 4-8 reps, no more than eight reps

- Lying Triceps Press. 2 sets, 6-10 reps

- Dumbbell Flyes. Three sets, 10 reps.

If your reading this book, you probably fall into the category of an endomorph. Having higher body fat composition and a tendency to store fat. Thus, losing weight is your main priority before building muscle. If you lose weight to FAST you could potentially get a condition called "loose skin," therefore do things in moderation. DO NOT rush. Loose skin is caused by losing huge amounts of weight (100+ lb.) in a short timeframe, and this creates disfiguring skin flaps. This usually happens when people do weight loss surgery as oppose to going the natural route, but there are some instances where people have gotten loose skin due to extremely fast weight loss through working out. Workout routine consists of rapid burst and short periods of rests, high-intensity interval training.

The intention here is doing as many workout reps as possible during a set time period.

Mesomorph is the most desired and favorable body type sought out after bodybuilders and athletes alike. Most athletes fall into the mesomorph continuum, and this particular body type excels extremely well in most mainstream sports because of its natural muscular build and dexterity that allows individuals to move quickly and be agile. Workouts consist of moderate to high-intensity interval training and short rest periods.

Importance of Gut Health- Probiotics

The gut can be considered your second brain and is where the majority of cells that make up your immune system are found. The entire digestive system has an important role to play in our health, ranging from the immune system, central nervous system, skin, blood pressure, and cardiovascular health.

The digestive system is composed of the stomach, small and large intestines, and other accessory organs. I want to specifically talk about the intestines as this is where the "good bacteria" are found. If you live anywhere in North America or any industrialized society for that matter, chances are you have poor gut health due to the wear and tear you've assaulted your body with from your lifestyle choices. From refined foods, alcohol, pollution, antibiotics, etc. You probably have a form of dysbiosis. -

Dysbiosis is just a fancy way of saying you have an imbalance of bacteria in your intestines.

Dysbiosis can manifest in many different forms, such as asthma, ear infections, excess mucous production in nose or throat, and even acne. When our gut is out of whack, it creates a domino effect throughout every significant system in the body. Thus, the importance of keeping our microbiome healthy because it is responsible for various essential physiological functions in our body, such as communicating with other cells, digestive processes, and detoxification of heavy metals, food toxins, and hormones by-products.

Hence, I stress the importance of consuming foods rich in probiotics too. Fermented food is where you can find loads of probiotics and fiber, which will aid in the repair and strengthening of your microbiome. The key to restoring gut health is 1. Eliminate food toxins 2. Use multiple strains of good bacteria 3. Consume more fiber.

Chapter 8: Keto Diet and Intermittent Fasting

Keto nutrition is a conventional nutritional treatment, established to remove the drawbacks of the non-conventional uses of fasting as management for epilepsy. In the 1920s and 1930s, this type of dieting witnessed its own abandonment. There was massive support of new anticonvulsant medicines. Many people who have epilepsy can effectively regulate their confiscations with drugs. But then again, around 30 percent of these patients are not able to control themselves even if they try various drugs. For the young people and kids precisely, the Keto Diet has found its way into the epilepsy world. Looking at the Keto Diet's history, you should emphasize on fasting, dieting, the decline of anticonvulsants, the MCT diet, and the revival of the Keto Diet.

Fasting: In ancient times, physicians used to cure certain diseases by interfering with their patient's meals. Epilepsy was considered as a supernatural disease in its origin as well as sure, and there was a proposal that nutritional treatment had a physical foundation. Some physicians claimed a possible cure of epilepsy as soon as it appeared through skipping of meals. The very first observation carried out in France in 1911, explaining that fasting was functional medicine for anyone with epilepsy was successful. The study involved 20 epilepsy patients and was of different ages. They were fed with foods with low fats, veggie diets, practiced together with some reasonable periods of fasting. Any epilepsy patient was to starve so that the disease can get cured. Fasting got popularized as a better method of restoring people's health. Many physicians recommended fasting for at least eighteen to twenty-five days to cure epilepsy. With a 90 percent water intake during the fasting period, many children and even young adults got cured of the epilepsy seizures. Therefore, fasting was recommended and practiced in conventional. Endocrinologists have reported their discovery that is treating epilepsy through starvation to the American Medical Association resolution. Even though fasting seemed a better medication for epilepsy, the seizures always returned after the fasting.

Dieting: Rollin Turner revised the study on diets and diabetes in 1921. He came to the conclusion that the liver produced three water molecules when they practiced fasting or when they consumed foods not rich in carbohydrates. Physicians, therefore, termed the 'Keto Diet' as nutrition that gave out increased levels of ketone molecules in the lifeblood after a high accumulation of calories and low levels of carbohydrates. Other physicians later formed 'the classic diet,' which involved rations of 1 gram of proteins for every kilogram of heaviness in children, ten to fifteen grams of carbohydrates daily, and the remaining fats from carbohydrates. There were positive effects associated with this type of dieting, that is, increased alertness, habits, and sleep. Unfavorable effects witnessed included vomiting caused by the significant amounts of ketone bodies. This type of dieting appeared favorable to the children as it improved seizure management on a diet. Though adults responded positively to the dieting as well, it was not as much as it did to the children.

The decline of anticonvulsants: Throughout the 1920 and 1930s, the keto diet was practiced, and that is the time where sedatives were the only anticonvulsant medicines available. However, this transformed when some doctors discovered new drugs, and every focus shifted on making more discoveries of new pills. By 1970, there were various drugs available to the doctors for the treatment of epileptic seizures, and this saw a decline in the usage of the keto diet as a medicine. Studies about the efficacy of the Keto diet declined until 1999, whereby the food was used to treat exceptional cases.

The MCT diet: Medium-chain triglycerides produced high levels of ketone molecules for every unit as compared to ordinary dietary calories. These triglycerides are easily absorbed and conveyed in the direction of the liver through the hepatic entryway system rather than the lymphatic coordination. The unembellished starch limitations made it hard for the parents to prepare appetizing diets which their kids would take, where approximately sixty percent of the fats came from the Medium-Chain Triglycerides. The MCT oil was then combined with skimmed milk and incorporated into the food: children with intractable seizures' health were improved through these diets.

The revival of the Keto diet: The Keto diet gained popularity in the United States of America in 1994 after Charlie Abraham's case was reported on NBC television. This young boy had uncontrollable epilepsy and did not get cured by any therapy that the doctors thought was the best. After practicing the keto diet, Charlie's average growth resumed. After Charlie's case was successfully treated, there were foundations aimed at studying more about this diet, and scientists began shifting their interests and focus on knowing more about the keto diet. By 2007, the keto diet had gained popularity in almost forty-five countries. Scientists and physicians concentrated on unleashing other possible uses of the keto diet rather than just treating epilepsy.

Keto diet's main aim is gaining more calories from proteins and oil rather than from carbohydrates. Your body's sugars get depleted, and this initiates fat breakdown, which leads to weight loss. But then again, the keto diet has its advantages and disadvantages, as discussed below.

Advantages of the Keto Diet

Helps in losing weight: Keto diet helps in burning fats into energy, and this fat breakdown leads to weight loss. The diet encourages high intake of proteins, and this ensures that you are not hungry most of the time during the fasting period. Out of the many ways of losing weight and fasting, the keto diet recorded the best results.

Helps reduce acne: Acne is caused by several factors, including the type of diet you take and the amount of sugar in your menus. Keto diet encourages eating foods that have fewer carbohydrates, and this helps reduce sugar levels, which helps maintain a healthy body and skin.

Reduces cancer risks

Recent studies conclude that keto diets can be used in the prevention of any chances of cancer. It may be used as an alternative treatment for radiation in people who have the disease. Just like intermittent fasting, keto diet causes increased oxidative stress in cells containing cancer as it does to the healthy cells. Keto diet reduces sugar levels in your blood, a factor that helps in lowering insulin levels, a hormone commonly associated with cancer.

Improves the health of the heart

Good adherence to the keto diet, for instance, taking natural fats such as avocadoes instead of meat, helps enhance the health of the center since it reduces cholesterol. Proper cholesterol levels are witnessed in keto diet observers.

Aids in brain functioning: Keto diet gives neuro-protective assistance, which helps prevent or even treat some brain-related illnesses such as sleep disorder. Children and young adults who do the keto diet always report high cognitive behaviors as well as alertness in their activities.

Reduces epilepsy seizures

If you mix calories, proteins, and carbohydrates, your body will change on how it uses its energy, leading to ketosis. Increased ketone molecules in the body help prevent epilepsy seizures, especially on children with focal seizures.

Advances the health of women suffering from PCOS

Polycystic Ovarian Syndrome is a specific illness that makes the ovaries to enlarge and have cysts. Studies show that taking foods rich in high carbohydrates could negatively impact women who suffer from PCOS. Though no detailed information about keto diet and PCOS, studies show that women who observe keto diet record massive weight loss, have their hormones balanced, have advanced luteinizing hormone, and have advanced starving insulin.

Disadvantages of a Keto Diet

Despite the above benefits, the keto diet has various shortcomings. Since the diet helps to cut the carbohydrates intake, this comes with several disadvantages as discussed below:

Keto flu: Various people report of falling sick immediately they start trying the keto diet. They associate this dieting with dizziness, vomiting, and weariness. But then again, this flu fades away as you get used to this dietary plan. About twenty-five percent of people who tried keto dietary reported having experienced this flu.

Fatigue was the most common factor. Physicians argue that people get flu because the body lacks enough sugar to breakdown as energy and uses fats instead. The solution to this is taking a lot of water and having enough sleep. You may also incorporate drinks like herbal tea or any adaptogenic herbs.

Diarrhea: Keto diet can make you run to the washrooms more often, and it is occasionally referred to as 'the keto diarrhea.' It is caused by the gallbladder, which is responsible for the production of bile, which helps in fat breakdown. Diarrhea can as well be caused by a lack of enough fiber in the body as this diet restricts carbohydrate intake.

The Keto Food Pills

Over the last years, there have been several signs of progress made to help understand the mechanisms of keto nutrition. On or after the multifaceted methodical, in addition to metabolic alterations brought by the keto diet, there have appeared the innovative hypotheses trying to connect organic versions to its experimental consequences. Regardless of such expansions, the important inquiry of how Keto nutrition operates continues being as indefinable as ever. In contemporary times, it is uncertain which of the various potential ways anticipated thus far are straight significant to the scientific consequences of the keto diet. It is improbable that these many suggestions can be amalgamated into a sole tool (or else a concluding mutual trail).

On the other hand, it may be educational to think through each one of these alleged devices in turn and enquire about the following query. On the condition that the procedure or objective in question is a life-threatening determining factor of the anticonvulsant effects of the keto nutrition, then would a comparable interference recognized to be grounded on that device produce an equivalent consequence? Conceivably responding to this query for each automatic assumption might assist validate (or overturn) that specific supposition. Can the keto diet be wrapped up into a tablet? At the moment, the response is likely to be a "no." Researchers have up till now to find out a "magical shot" that wholly reflects the anticonvulsant (as well as possible neuro-protective) impacts of the keto nutrition.

Scientists in the ketogenic nutrition (KD) field of study have similarly included these codes of belief and in recent times, boarded on that all-too-conversant quixotic passage, with the final purpose of decreasing the "problematic" keto nutrition procedure to a modest pill. If this is attained, the consequence will portray a sarcastic restatement of the initial past of the keto regime in the USA.

Even though the keto food went through an early flow of attention succeeding its beginning in the first 1920s, the diet was reduced in importance to close insignificance through the appearance of a familiar medication identified as the phonation. From this time forth, up until the middle of the 1990s, doctors – for understandable, practical whys and wherefores – found it unassuming to recommend a tablet instead of challenging nutrition.

First Conception: It is probably GABA!

A lot of the current anticonvulsant medicines put forth consequences on restraint Neuro-transmission, also extra unambiguously, by means of improving the synaptic intensities of amino-butyric sourness known as GABA or else moderating post-synaptic GABAA receptors. Cases in point of such go-betweens consist of molecules such as tiagabine, vigabatrin, benzodiazepines, barbiturates, felbamate, and topiramate. As a result, granted the riches of statistics on the subject of GABA-ergic neurotransmission, one likelihood is that the keto diet, conceivably via the ketone builds, maybe answerable for uplifting synaptic heights of GABA that would then produce an inhibitory (in addition the hypothetical anticonvulsant) outcome.

Studies circulated widely have demonstrated the effects of the ketone molecules on wits glutamate plus GABA metabolism. One study, in particular, indicated that adding up of both aceto-acetate and β-hydroxyl-butyrate improved the development of branded GABA and was also associated with reduced intake of glutamate through trans-amination to aspartate. A similar study had presented that Ketone bodies improve the amalgamation of GABA in synaptic-stones extracted from rodent forebrain.

Consequently, one primary arising question is if ketone supplements influence inhibitory (otherwise excitatory) neurotransmission? Inopportunely, the response is that (no less than now) thoughtfully decisive study is poised on the concept that severe claim of BHB in addition to ACA did not impact some characteristics. In addition, if the keto diet rises GABA intensities in wits, then that consequence is estimated through vigabatrin, an irreparable restrictor of the unoriginal "enzyme GABA trans-aminase," and by tiagabine, GABA re-approval restrictor that restricts with pre-synaptic GABA transmitters. The anti-convulsing profile of the Keto Diet is different from that of vigabatrin plus tiagabine. The all-purpose method of originating one more medication that improves brain GABA points might not be pertinent or feasible, from the time when many confiscation kinds appear to be worsened by representatives that lead to improved refreshment inhibition, and extra-synaptic GABA receptors that intercede stimulant inhibition are extra-penetrating to raise encompassing GABA attentions. Without a doubt, improved GABA-ergic reticence in cortex looks as if it lies beneath the contrivance of bringing together confiscation group in two mouse representations of auto-somal prevailing night-time anterior section epileptic condition.

Second Conception: Acetone plus Aceto-acetate!

The most primitive protest of unswerving in vivo consequences of ketone figures was prepared by researchers during the 1930s, while the conclusion was that aceto-acetate when ordered intraperitoneally in bunnies, disallowed confiscations. It is a convulsing integral evident in numerous vital oils and an opponent of GABAA receptors. That influential remark was far ahead of established in an audiogenic confiscation-susceptible mouse classical. Interestingly, researchers have established that the comprehensive anticonvulsant assets of acetone in 4 dissimilar living thing systems, plus when vaccinated intraperitoneally, created plasma and Cerebra-Spinal Fluid attentions reliable with the ones that tended to overpower confiscations. The consequences established and prolonged chronological explanations backing up an anticonvulsant deed for acetone finished as yet undecided contrivances.

And in advance sustenance of this, the further inquiry found that acetone was measurable (capable of inattentiveness of 0.7 mm) in the psychological ability of a patient with epilepsy by expending proton. Granted these explanations, would it be concrete to wrap up aceto-acetate or acetone into a medication? Despite the fact that the fact ketone supplements are expected to affect the indigenous of cellular bioenergetics, there are thoughtful logistical constrictions that are preventing the ease of managing persons to accomplish similar low milli-molar absorptions experimented in scientific explorations. The stability of aceto-acetate is evidently inherent in its instant inclination to instructively decarboxylase, and acetone is a renowned solvent that can lead to important mucosal discomfort. To that end, oral absorption of β-hydroxyl-butyrate preparations to achieve this type of intake may not be objectively and fundamentally attainable. These contemplations positions are not minor encounters with the intention of a ketone medication. One of the irritating unsettled inquiries concerning ketone figures is whether they relate to the inhibition regulator. Contemporary studies have recommended that under a number of circumstances and in precise representations, blood points of ketones do not join well with anticonvulsant outcomes. On the other hand, ketone points are recognized to differ significantly all through the diurnal sequence, characteristically as a result of eating patterns and the succeeding breakdown of food substances. Regardless of abundant studies emphasizing ketonemia as being behind the Keto Diet cure, it is still not known what exactly defines the right brain attentions, particularly in the small environment of the tremendously broken-down lively synapse. Furthermore, other researches are signifying that increased ketone figure intensities are not essential for experimental effectiveness of an increased-fat diet in contradiction to medically headstrong epilepsies.

Third Conception: Intensification in Bioenergetics

A single potential description for the anticonvulsant accomplishment of the Keto Diet contends that augmented ATP combination should yield a confident bioenergetics equilibrium, letting steadying of the inactive film possible through the improved activities of

Na+-K+-ATPase. More than a few years ago, some researchers described that the Keto Diet enlarged the total number of bioenergetics substrates (for instance, adenosine triphosphate, or ATP) and raised the liveliness charge. These ups and downs were alleged to alleviate the cell thickness, mainly in the expression of unnecessary excitation. Unswerving with these explanations, a progressive human study applying magnetic reverberation spectroscopic methods showed that people with epilepsy who nourished a keto regime had raised phosphor-creatine up to creatine points in wits. In recent times, by means of the cDNA microarray know-how, enlarged appearance of the "mitochondrial ATP synthase β," D sub-unit in a rat's mind was conveyed following keto nutrition cure. And in the greatest complete research of that form to the current time, the keto diet was discovered to improve "mitochondrial biogenesis" plus meaningfully enhance the quantity of genetic factors in mice. That enhancement in bioenergetics ability empowered "hippocampal" parts of the rats to endure better the metabolic task of operating on little glucose experience.

Consequently, is the experimental efficiency of the keto diet merely an issue of accumulating fuel stocks? On the condition that this is the situation, then would the situation not become a more upfront issue to consume creatine, an extremely bioavailable and comparatively secure oral enhancement that is more and more established to encourage physical condition and durability?

Fourth Conception: Reducing Sensitive Oxygen Kinds

It is soundly recognized that any intensification in "mitochondrial film potential ($\triangle \psi$) can promote mitochondrial reactive oxygen species (ROS) generation through increased electron pushing. Mitochondrial uncoupling proteins (UCPs) – which are activated by fatty acids – increase proton conductance and dissipate $\triangle \psi$, thereby decreasing ROS formation. Recent studies have implicated UCPs as potential mediators of a neuroprotective effect of the KD". Furthermore, "the UCP2 expression" in trans-genic rat decreased confiscation-stimulated neural cells and is successively linked with improved ATP intensities and reduced ROS releasing. The high fat-suckling practice in normal pests is a defensive counter to kainite-persuaded neuronal demise in undeveloped rat hippocampus. This is a consequence that was accredited to the oily acid-persuaded intensifications in UCP2 appearance and a decrease in ROS making.

And as a final point, the keto diet cure in standard young mice steered to improved hippocampal appearance and movement of all three acknowledged mind-localizable isoforms of UCP (that is, UCP2, UCP4, plus UCP5), and connected with important reductions in ROS intensities." As a consequence, on condition that fatty bitterness (plus possibly extra suitably, poly-unsaturated oily acid otherwise PUFA), improve the mitochondrial disengagement, and on the condition that this fundamental down-stream device is accountable for both the anti-convulsing as well as neuroprotective impacts (they have hitherto to be established), then can getting a biochemical un-intertwine for instance "2, 4-dinitrophenol (DNP)" produce similar results? Unquestionably, it is better acknowledged that this chemical, a compelling mitochondrial un-intertwine that intensely upsurges the fat breakdown speed, and on different instances applied to cure corpulence during the 1930s, obligates an important unfortunate side-effect profile; in precision, these effects are a high infection and the danger of death. Fewer toxic compounds are essential when there is a mitochondrial disconnection.

Fifth Conception: Improving Glutathione

Even as the connection amid the seizure movement, the oxidative pressure, and the neuronal damage presently do not seem to be explained, past examinations by researchers have demonstrated that imperfections in cell reinforcement frameworks "may add to seizure beginning and epileptogenesis." Are there different components by which the oxidative pressure can be constricted in the epileptic cerebrum? Glutathione refers to an endogenous tri-peptide cancer prevention agent whose capacity is to forestall liberated radical-intervened cell damage; it is present in every cell within the human body, and solely in its decreased structure "(GSH)" because of the compressive action of "glutathione reductase" which changes it from its oxidized condition, "glutathione disulfide (GSSG)." In states of oxidative pressure, The "glutathione reductase" can subsequently lead to increase the decreasing reciprocals that are essential for eliminating apprehensive elements, for example receptive oxygen. In rodents stimulated in a KD, there was a growth in cancer prevention agent action utilizing a luminal oxidation measure in the hippocampus and a four-crease increment in glutathione peroxidase movement. Steady with these discoveries, researchers of late have detailed an up-guideline of GSH biosynthesis in youthful rodents bolstered with Keto Diet.

Moreover, these scholars watched the improved mitochondrial cell reinforcement status and suggested that the progressions were as a result of avoiding mitochondrial DNA from oxidant-initiated harm. By and large, these examinations recommend that the KD may, for sure, apply neuroprotective action. All in all, in the event that the KD demonstrations mainly to upgrade glutathione levels in the cerebrum, at that point, would take glutathione enhancements (that are financially accessible) be adequate to ensure in opposition to abduction movement? The appropriate response is negative given that available glutathione plans are processed prior to getting into the circulatory system, let unaccompanied to the cerebrum. The main enhancement that successfully brings glutathione to step up in the body is "N-acetyl-L-cysteine (NAC)," which has generally been utilized to cure liver harmfulness incited by dangerous degrees of acetaminophen. Therefore, would NAC be an appropriate alternative for the Keto Diet? The scientific knowledge to the present time has been blended, with certain persons with dynamic myoclonic epilepsies enhancing NAC alternation.

Sixth Conception: Dropping Glycolysis Plus Calorie Limitation?

The reduction of glycolysis is regarded as the key system of KD activity. The prevalence of seizure is lessened by calorie limitation in rodents, and the resulting decreased blood sugar intensifications associated with the hindrance of epileptogenesis in a hereditary form of boost instigated epilepsy. Along related lines, studies have exhibited that seizures were concentrated seizure movement in rodents due to the hindrance of the glycolytic catalyst phosphor-glucose by 2-deoxyglucose, and similarly diminished the outflow of cerebrum inferred "neurotrophic factor (BDNF)" and its foremost recipient, the TrkB.

In the recent times, explorations have showed that "fructose-1, 6-bisphosphate (F-1, 6-BP)", a metabolite that moves the digestion of sugar from "glycolysis to the pentose phosphate pathway, displays intense anticonvulsant action" in a few rodent forms of intense confiscations (that is, "pilocarpine, kainic corrosive, and pentylenetetrazole"), and viability in these forms surpasses that of "2-DG and KD treatment". All things considered, this developing information demonstrates that the general system of restricting glycolytic transition might be an incredible method for anticipating intense seizures and maybe epileptogenesis also. One inquiry remarkably examined component ensnared in the scientific advantages of calorie limitation includes sirtuins, a huge and assorted group of chemicals that manage quality articulation. The first sirtuin was successively portrayed in mildew; "Sir2 is a class III histone deacetylase that uses the cofactor nicotinamide adenine dinucleotide (NAD+)" in synergist response that discharges nicotinamide (a criticism inhibitor) and "O-acetyl ADP ribose."

It has been accounted for that expanded Sir2 action protracts life expectancy, and that calorie confinement builds "Sir2 levels" and does not advance life span in "SIR2 knockouts".

In well-evolved creatures, calorie limitation expands the statement of "Sirt1", the "Sir2" mammalian ortholog, in different body tissues, together with the mind. "Resveratrol", is a component present in red wine (scientific name "activator Sirt1"), of the research carried out on mice, have shown that this component extends life expectancy and makes the decay of the motor work for the year expire.

AMP kinase action in the neurons is animated by resveratrol, and additionally critically, ensures against kainic corrosive initiated seizures and oxidative anxiety in rodents. Along these lines, if resveratrol, an eating regimen determined nutraceutical, can reproduce the impacts of calorie confinement, diminish oxidative pressure, and ensure against seizure action, at that point drinking red wine, which contains resveratrol, is an excellent habit that can be incorporated into the daily food routine by combining it with the indications provided by a nutritionist or any specialists dealing with the nervous system. In the clinical setting, all persons cured with the Keto nutrition are below the lawful age for taking alcohol, and additionally, liquor utilization at early times – regardless of whether upheld for restoratively headstrong epilepsy – might cause "apoptotic neuro-degeneration." Then again, if straightforward calories confinement is adequate to avert seizure movement in persons, why not diminish absolute caloric admission, and not mess with the high-fat Keto Diet? In the event that it is so, from a different point of view, one could think about consolidating the Keto Diet and calorie limitation (as has been accomplished in creature ponders). In rodents encouraged a calories-confined Keto Diet, research demonstrated that increasingly huge combined heartbeat hindrance in the dentate gyrus, raised maximal dentate enactment limit. These outcomes propose that a cure with a calorie-limited KD may create both anticonvulsant and against epileptogenic impacts.

Seventh Conception: Leaping Towards Leptin

Leptin is a fundamental protein hormone that basically manages vitality admission and use. The components through which leptin applies its impacts on digestion are, for the most part, obscure. Despite the fact that leptin is prevalently originating from adipocytes, it is additionally found exceptionally transmitted in territories of the nerve center. Curiously, leptin balances various film bound particle channels and applies differential consequences for neuronal sensitivity. The importance of leptin to seizure defenselessness was as of late featured by who exhibited a fundamentally diminished edge in "leptin-insufficient ob/ob mice to pentylenetetrazol-instigated seizures. Certainly, leptin itself restrains seizures instigated by 4-aminopyridine and pentylenetetrazole-actuated", conceivably through the bar of AMPA receptor-interceded synaptic transmission. In the event that the constraining of AMPA receptor-interceded transmission is a basic factor, it ought to be reviewed; this can likewise be cultivated by topiramate. Regarding the Keto Diet, the leptin flagging framework is accepted to add to the moderate weight increase related to ceaseless treatment in the two rodents. Higher serum leptin levels and lower insulin levels were found in Keto Diet-bolstered adolescent rodents than control rodents. While the impacts of leptin on seizure weakness and its relationship to Keto Diet-initiated weight reduction are fascinating, currently there exists no information that can support the mediatory role of leptin as an anticonvulsant of the Keto Diet. To be specific on the issue of some fascinating recent research, intranasal organization of leptin may be proficient in prematurely ending intense seizure action. Also, if the clinical impacts of the Keto Diet are expected to a limited extent to expanded leptin levels, at that point, quickened improvement and approval of leptin as a novel anticonvulsant drug would be justified.

Eighth Conception: Poly-unsaturated Fatty Acids

Polyunsaturated unsaturated fats (PUFAs, for example, "docosahexaenoic corrosive (DHA, C22: 6ω-3), arachidonic corrosive (AA, C20: 4ω-3), or eicosapentaenoic corrosive (EPA, C20: 5ω-3) have been accounted for stifling voltage-gated sodium channels, and L-type calcium diverts in seizure-inclined structures", for example, the hippocampus. The Keto Diet produces heights of both AA and DHA in the serum of patients and animals, separately, recommending that these substrates may apply anticonvulsant impacts by restraining sodium and calcium channels, in the same way as other anticonvulsant drugs. Given these discoveries, it isn't amazing that researchers have contemplated the impacts of dietary supplementation with PUFAs alone, to decide if these substrates can render an anticonvulsant impact. Early case reports proposed that this methodology is able to control and manage seizures appropriately. In any case, an ongoing randomized preliminary in grown-up patients with epilepsy neglected to exhibit the predominance of a PUFA supplement "(EPA) in addition to DHA, 2.2 mg/day in a 3:2 proportion." In this manner, the research is still continuing to determine whether PUFAs alone can reflect the clinical impacts of the Keto Diet.

Ninth Conception: It Is a Touch of Everything

Over the previous decade, research shows that an assortment of atomic, hereditary, cell, and metabolic components are likely contributory to the clinical impacts of the Keto Diet. As a speculation, it is getting to be acknowledged that the robotic underpinnings of the Keto Diet are sensible numerous, parallel, and potentially synergistic. So, the inquiry remains, can the Keto Diet be bundled into a pill? At this stage, given our condition of information, the presumable answer is NO! At that point, we might be able to adopt a polypharmacy strategy and build up a few prescriptions, each with an unmistakable robotic target? Such a technique would not be excessively the same as what is rehearsed by grown-ups – and particularly, the older – who are by both need and decision on multi-tranquilize regimens and multi-wholesome enhancements, again to accomplish wellbeing and avoid the attacks of maturing and illness. There is likely no "enchantment slug" that totally reflects the anticonvulsant (and "potential neuroprotective") impacts of the Keto Diet; the equivalent could be said for the treatment of the epilepsies, "a gathering of related conditions with broadly unique etiologies," and consequently a variety of basic pathophysiological components. Presently, without inquiring about the complex metabolic riddle presented by the Keto Diet, we would again be left with just subjective perceptions, and to wonder thoughtfully how a high-fat eating regimen can apply such significant clinical impacts.

What to Expect on a Keto Diet

Therapeutic specialists have used ketogenic or keto supper plans for almost 100 years to deal with certain ailments. In any case, as of late, the high-fat, low-starch eating style has turned out to be well known among competitors, wellness aficionados, and individuals hoping to get thinner. On the off chance that you choose to go on a keto diet, you can hope to roll out considerable improvements to your eating style. This eating regimen wipes out or seriously limits numerous nourishments that you are likely used to eating.

What You Should Eat

The ketogenic diet, or keto nutrition, is an inadequate sugar eating plan that powers the body to utilize fat instead of glucose as an essential vitality source. When you pursue the technique, you make suppers around fatty nourishments, and this essentially limits your intake of starch and protein nutrients. Because of that macronutrients steadiness, ketones (these acids) are created in the body. At the point when the ketone levels are sufficiently high, you are in a condition of ketosis. Preparing your body into (and remaining in) a condition of ketosis is the objective of a keto diet. While no particular sustenance is beyond reach, you will experience considerable difficulties, incorporating numerous basic nourishments in your supper arrangement when you are attempting to come to the macronutrient steadiness that is necessary.

Acceptable Food Items

- Dairy Products
- Poultry
- Oily shellfish and fish
- Low-carbohydrate vegetables
- Plant-based oils
- Olives, nuts, plus seeds
- Avocado, margarine, nutty spread

Rebellious Foods

- Generally organic product
- Overcast or high fiber vegetables
- Grains items, for example, bread, pasta, or heated products
- Beans and lentils
- Complete grains (like quinoa, farro, wheat) and rice
- Sugar refreshments and generally liquor
- Delicacy or sweet pastries

Consistent Foods

Full Fat Dairy: Dairy items, for example, eggs, most cheddar, margarine, and sizeable cream, are utilized for cooking and are part of the different plans for cuisine. Full fat curds, notorious yogurt, and whole milk are additionally used.

Poultry: Chicken and turkey can get incorporated into suppers on the keto diet. Dim meat is favored in light of the fact that it will, in general, be higher in fat. Additionally, dim meat, (for example, thighs and legs) is progressively top in myoglobin—oxygen-conveying protein.

Oily Fish: Fresh fish can offer you an opportunity to make dinner. Assortments, for example, salmon or fish, are high in heart-sound omega-3 unsaturated fats. Shellfish, mussels, shrimp, and scallops and fish are additionally protein sources that you ought to devour on a keto diet.

Low-Carbohydrate Vegetables: Some vegetables are low in carbs as a nutrient even though they are high in fiber and vitamins, some are low enough in carbs to be incorporated into a keto supper plan. These include vegetables like asparagus, cucumber, kale, tomato, eggplant, and spinach.

Plant-Based Oils: Individuals importing the keto diet plans consistently use oils to expand their fat admission. Coconut oil and other plant-based oils contain medium-chain triglycerides (MCTs), which nutritiously important. MCTs are immediately assimilated and are accepted to help get the body into ketosis. Other plant-based oils include oil from these plants; sesame avocado oil, and olive.

Olives, Nuts, and Seeds: In a keto diet, snack nourishments should come in plenty. Individuals following the arrangement by and large use nuts and seeds that contain a modest quantity of protein and solid fat. Pumpkin seeds, chia seeds, almond seeds are a favorite, alongside olives.

Butter, Avocado, and Peanut Butter: Individuals following the keto diet don't regularly utilize spreads since they don't devour bread or wafers. Whenever butter is used, margarine and avocado are top decisions. Peanut butter can be similarly consumed just in case it does not contain sugar.

Resistant Foods

Most Fruit: A fruit is an important source of both fiber and glucose. Since naturally occurring fruits are rich in fiber, vitamin, and folic acid, they are not appropriate for consumption in a keto diet. It should be noted that a number of individuals can eat limited quantities of berries (for example, raspberries) and still remain in ketosis.

Low or Fiber-Rich Vegetables: Vegetables that include sweet potatoes, onions, beets, carrots, potatoes, and peas are by and large stayed away from as they contain an excessive amount of sugar and such significant quantities of carbs.

Grains and Grain Products: Large quantities of starch and fiber are obtained from grains and grain products. This includes items such as whole grains, including quinoa, farro, and wheat, that give the keto diet high amounts of fiber and starch. Likewise, items that are made from grains or grain products are not included in the keto plans. Rice, rice items, and nibble sustenance (chips, pretzels, and saltines) should never be suggested in keto diet; these food items are usually lower in fiber, yet high in starch (another type of sugar).

Beans and Lentils: Beans, lentils, peanuts, peas, and different kinds of vegetables consumed by vegetarians to supplement their protein intake and requirements are a rich source of protein. Despite that, these nutritious foodstuffs are not incorporated on ketogenic diet since they give an excessively large amount of starch, just like fiber.

Alcoholic drinks and Sugary Beverages: Soft drinks, tea, sports drinks, and juice are typically a significant source of sugar in a normal American diet. These beverages are not prompted on the keto diet since they include starch without giving any significant supplements. Zero-calorie sugars are likewise not prescribed in light of the fact that they can build your yearnings for desserts.

By and large, liquor isn't prompted. However, some keto supporters drink low-carb drinks with some limitations. For instance, taking hard beverages (counting rum, vodka, gin, tequila, and bourbon) gives zero grams of starch. Wine, for the most part, contains around 3–4 grams of carb per serving. Most lager is high in carbs and is maintained at a strategic distance from the keto diet.

Treat and Dessert

As you may guess, candy and other sweet treats are not part of the keto diet. Most customary treats are high in fat yet additionally high in sugar. Despite the fact that counterfeit sugars are commonly not suggested, a few people following a keto diet make fat bombs and different treats utilizing keto-explicit heating items, for example, extraordinarily checking confectioners' sugar and chocolate chips.

Prescribed Planning

There is no particular planning and timing that is required when observing a ketogenic diet. A large number of people keep up an ordinary time plan as their eating style. In any case, a few people on the ketogenic diet practice discontinuous fasting and either skirt a feast during the day or just eat during explicit spaces of time opening up during the day. In the event that you eat three meals daily, then these dietary plans will give you a thought of what eating a keto diet resembles. In the event that you are thinking about the ketogenic diet, you can assess every day's meal and consider whether the sustenance is satisfactorily enough, and if the eating style appears to be sensible.

Keto Diet Plan

Keto plan originates from tourists and athletes who use the eating style to improve their gaming exercise. Patrick Sweeney likewise addresses the ketogenic diet through conferences he attends around the world, encouraging individuals to try the plan providing them with a personal experience. His example of a dietary plan is simple and fantastic for persons who like to cook.

Keto Diet First Day

Breakfast: Adventure espresso (an extraordinary formula that joins espresso with coconut oil, substantial cream, butter, an egg, and at times cocoa powder) alone, or include breakfast cheddar blintzes. Blend a cup of cream cheddar with three egg whites in a blender. Include cream powder and smoked salmon or crisp berries when preparing the blintzes like flapjacks, at that point, include cream cheddar and smoked salmon or crisp raspberries.

Early in the day nibble: Full-fat Greek yogurt

Lunch: Serving of mixed greens with either of these food items salmon, chicken, or barbecued shrimp and cheddar.

Evening nibble: Apple with almond margarine

Supper: Grilled salmon, cauliflower, spinach, or green beans heated with smashed cheddar.

Pastry: One square of dim (>72 percent cacao) chocolate

Keto Diet Second Day

Breakfast: Escapade espresso alone or include a fountain of liquid magma eggs. Whip two egg whites to standing and then top with a couple of spinach leaves and a bit of smoked salmon. Spread cheddar on top and make a hole in the top with a spoon. Prepare for 5 minutes at 350F at that point, but the burden in the indent, and let it shower down the seared sides.

Early in the day nibble: Goat's milk yogurt with a bunch of almonds

Lunch: Goat cheddar serving of mixed greens with pecans and bacon

Evening nibble: Almonds

Supper: Turkey stew with beans, onions, tomatoes, peppers, and ground cheddar. Discretionary: include a broiled egg top. Eat with a side plate of mixed greens.

Keto Diet Third Day

Breakfast: Adventure espresso alone or with an additional thick omelet. Sauté garlic, cherry tomatoes, red and green peppers, and avocado in a skillet. When they are delicately cooked, take them out, including olive oil, and blend in two eggs for an omelet. Include your preferred cheddar and fresh spinach.

A bite in the morning: Apple with butter spread

Lunch: Leftover food items from the earlier night

Evening bite: Brie and a Wasa saltine (an exceptionally low starch wafer)

Supper: Duck on the grill with flame-broiled eggplant and zucchini

Macro-nutrient steadiness

Sonny, during his start of a ketogenic diet plan, does not adhere to a particular macronutrient balance. Rather, he keeps up an eating routine that incorporates close to 50 grams of starch every day. When he goes over 0.6 on the ketone meter (a gadget used to gauge blood for the nearness of ketones), he goes as much as 70 grams of sugars and takes a ketone supplement. Ketone enhancements are accepted to help fat cells to functionally separate adequately, despite the fact that the science to help their utilization is inadequate.

Chapter 9: Recipes

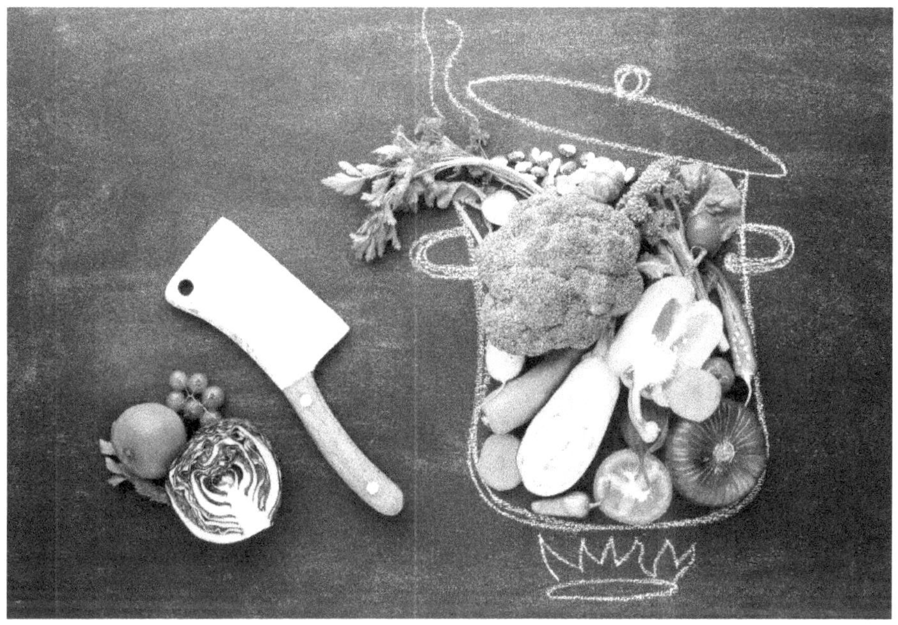

Now it's time to see how to prepare delicious meals using the ketogenic diet for intermittent fasting!

Breakfast Menu Options

Bacon & Avocado Omelet

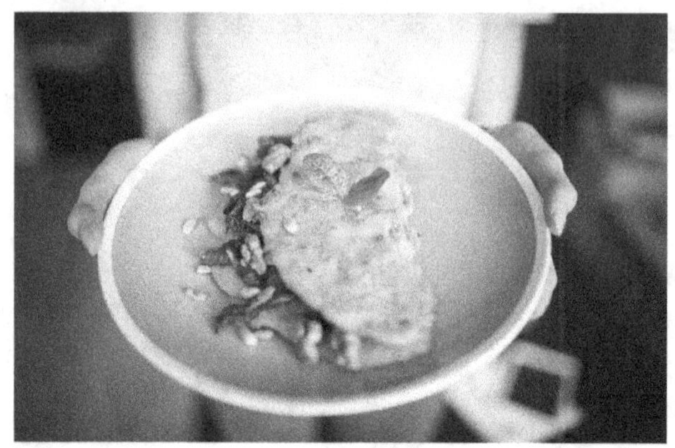

Yields Provided: 1 serving

Prep & Cook Time: 10 minutes

Nutritional Value Per Serving:

•	**Calorie Counts**	•	719
•	**Net Carbohydrates**	•	3.3 grams
•	**Protein**	•	30 grams
•	**Total Fats**	•	63 grams

Ingredients:

- Crispy bacon (1 slice)
- Parmesan cheese (.5 cup)
- Large eggs (2)
- Ghee/coconut oil/butter (2 tbsp.)
- Salt (1 pinch)
- Small avocado (half of 1)

Prep Technique:

1. Prepare the bacon as desired and set aside.
2. Grate and combine the parmesan cheese, eggs, and your choice of finely chopped herbs.
3. Warm a skillet and add the butter to melt using the med-high temperature setting.
4. When the pan is hot, whisk and add the eggs.
5. Prepare the omelet working it towards the middle of the pan for about 30 seconds. When firm, flip it over and cook for another 30 seconds.
6. Arrange on a plate and garnish with the crunched bacon bits. Serve with sliced avocado.

Blueberry Hemp Seed Breakfast Oatmeal

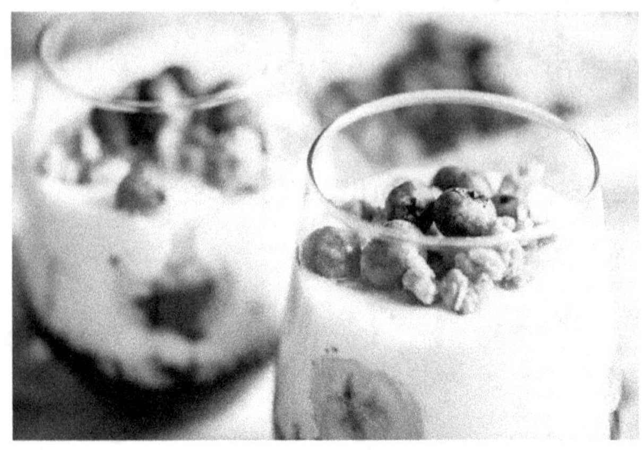

Yields Provided: 2 servings

Prep & Cook Time: 10 minutes

Nutritional Value Per Serving:

•	**Calorie Counts**	•	436
•	**Net Carbohydrates**	•	5 grams
•	**Protein**	•	21 grams
•	**Total Fats**	•	31 grams

Ingredients:

- Unsweetened almond milk/water (1 cup)
- Ground cinnamon (.5 tsp.)
- Hemp seed hearts (.5 cup)
- Flaxseed meal (.5 cup)
- Swerve (2 tbsp.)
- Unsweetened coconut flakes (1 tbsp.)
- Fresh blueberries (.25 cup)
- Vanilla extract (1 tsp.)
- Sliced almonds (1 tbsp.)

Prep Technique:

1. Place a saucepan over the med-high heat using the stovetop. Pour in the milk, vanilla extract, and cinnamon. Stir.
2. Toss in the hemp seed hearts and flaxseed meal. Change the temperature on the stove to medium heat.
3. Stir in the sweetener. Keep the mixture on the heat (uncovered) until the oatmeal thickens.
4. Serve in a bowl and top with almonds, blueberries, and other keto-friendly toppings.

Cocoa Waffles

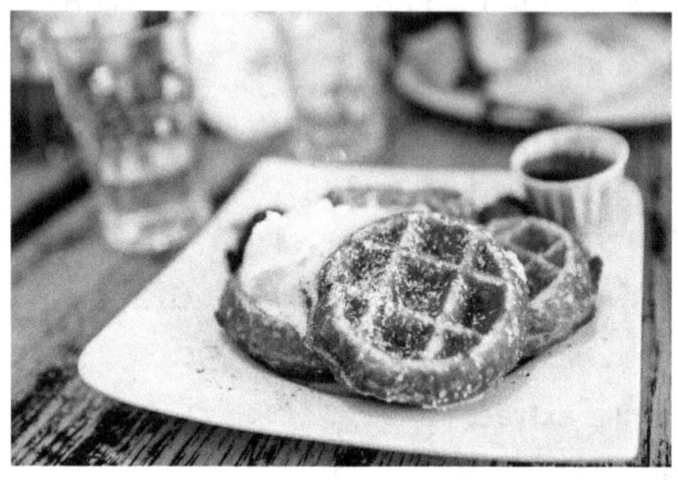

Yields Provided: 5 servings

Prep & Cook Time: 35 minutes

Nutritional Value Per Serving:

•	**Calorie Counts**	•	289
•	**Net Carbohydrates**	•	3.4 grams
•	**Protein**	•	7 grams
•	**Total Fats**	•	27 grams

Ingredients:

- Separated eggs (5)
- Unsweetened cocoa (.25 cup)
- Granular sweetener (3 tbsp.)
- Coconut flour (4 tbsp.)
- Baking powder (1 tsp.)
- Melted butter (4.5 oz.)
- Milk of choice (3 tbsp.)
- Vanilla (1 tsp.)

Prep Technique:

1. Use a whisk to prepare the egg whites. Briskly mix to form stiff peaks.
2. In another container, whisk the sweetener, baking powder, and cocoa with the egg yolks.
3. Add the butter to the dry mixture. Stir in vanilla and milk.
4. Fold in the prepared egg whites a little at a time.
5. Transfer the mixture in the waffle maker.
6. Cook until they are golden brown.
7. Serve.

Ham & Cheese Soufflé

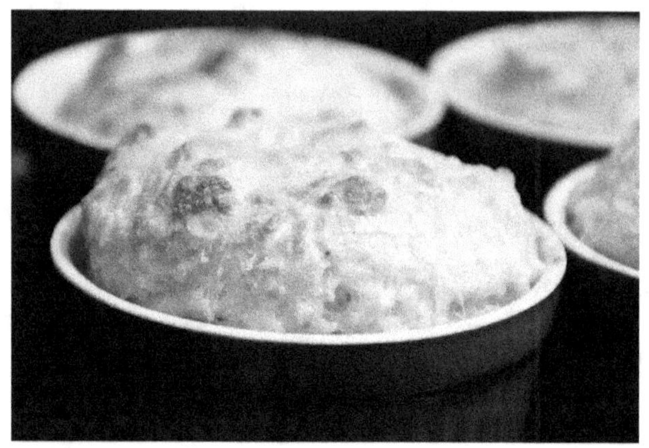

Yields Provided: 4 servings

Prep & Cook Time: 30-35 minutes

Nutritional Value Per Serving:

• **Calorie Counts**	•	460
• **Net Carbohydrates**	•	5 grams
• **Protein**	•	24 grams
• **Total Fats**	•	38 grams

Ingredients:

- Diced yellow onion (1 small)
- Minced garlic (2 cloves)
- Fresh chopped chives (2 tbsp.)
- Shredded cheddar cheese (1 cup)
- Heavy cream (.5 cup)
- Eggs (6 large)
- Diced ham (6 oz.)
- Salt and pepper (as desired)
- Olive oil (2 tbsp.)
- Also Needed: 6 oz. ramekins (4)

Prep Technique:

1. Program the oven setting to reach 400° Fahrenheit. Lightly grease the ramekins.
2. Use the medium heat temperature setting in a skillet on the stovetop to warm the oil.
3. Toss in the onions to sauté for five minutes. Next, toss in the garlic and sauté for one more minute.
4. Whisk together the rest of the fixings in a mixing bowl.

5. Add the cooked onions and garlic. Stir
    well, then divide among the ramekins.
6. Bake until the egg is cooked through (18
    to 22 minutes).
7. Cool slightly before serving.

Sausage Hot Pockets

Yields Provided: 2 servings

Prep & Cook Time: 30-35 minutes

Nutritional Value Per Serving:

•	**Calorie Counts**	•	510
•	**Net Carbohydrates**	•	6.6 grams
•	**Protein**	•	26.3 grams
•	**Total Fats**	•	41.4 grams

Ingredients:

- Low-moisture shredded mozzarella cheese (.75 cup)
- Almond flour (.33 cup)
- Egg white (1)
- *Optional:* Xanthan gum (.5 tsp.)
- *The Filling:*
- Shredded Mexican blend cheese
- Avocado oil (1 tbsp.)

- Large eggs (2)
- Kiolbassa Jalapeno Smoked Sausage (1)
- Bell pepper (2 tbsp.)
- Jalapeno pepper (1 tbsp.)
- Onion (2 tbsp.)

Prep Technique:

1. Heat the oven to reach 400° Fahrenheit.
2. Melt the cheese in the microwave for about 30 seconds.
3. Stir in the rest of the fixings. Roll into a ball, kneading one or two times.
4. Place the ball between two sheets of parchment baking paper. With a rolling pin, prepare the dough to a .25-inch thickness.
5. Warm oil in a cast-iron skillet using the med-high heat setting.
6. Once it is hot, add in onions and peppers to simmer for two or three minutes until softened.
7. Stir in the sausage, cooking for another 2 to 3 minutes. Push aside and add the eggs. Scramble until done.

8. Place the mixture into the center of the dough. Tuck in each of the sides until fully enclosed. Poke with a fork for the steam to escape.

9. Bake for 20 minutes. Remove and slice in half to serve.

Lunch Menu Options

Salad Choices

Caprese Salad

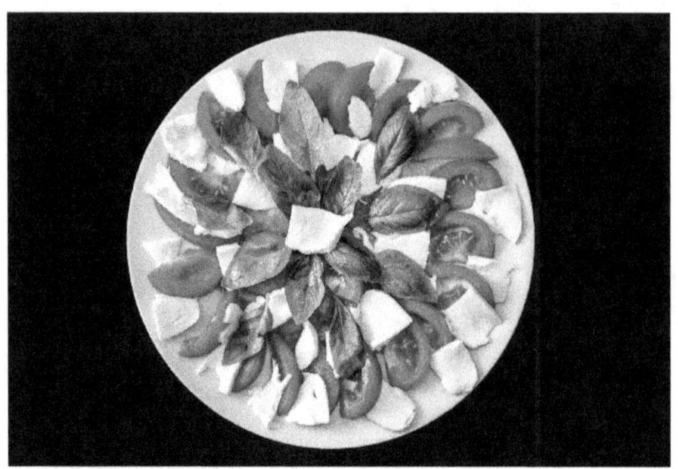

Yields Provided: 4 servings

Prep & Cook Time: 40 minutes

Nutritional Value Per Serving:

•	**Calorie Counts**	•	191
•	**Net Carbohydrates**	•	5 grams
•	**Protein**	•	8 grams

• **Total Fats**	• 64 grams

Ingredients:

- Grape tomatoes (3 cups)
- Peeled garlic cloves (4)
- Avocado oil (2 tbsp.)
- Mozzarella balls (19 pearl-sized)
- Baby spinach leaves (4 cups)
- Brine reserved from the cheese (1 tbsp.)
- Pesto (1 tbsp.)
- Fresh basil leaves (.25 cup)

Prep Technique:

1. Use a layer of foil to line a baking tray.
2. Set the oven temperature setting to 400º Fahrenheit.
3. Arrange the cloves and tomatoes on the baking pan and drizzle using the oil. Bake until the tops are lightly browned (20-30 min.).
4. Drain the liquid from the mozzarella (saving one tablespoon). Mix the pesto with the brine.
5. Rinse and drain the spinach before adding to a large salad bowl. Transfer the tomatoes to the

dish along with the roasted garlic. Drizzle with the pesto sauce.

6. Garnish with the mozzarella balls and freshly torn basil leaves.

Cauliflower Rice Salad - Instant Pot

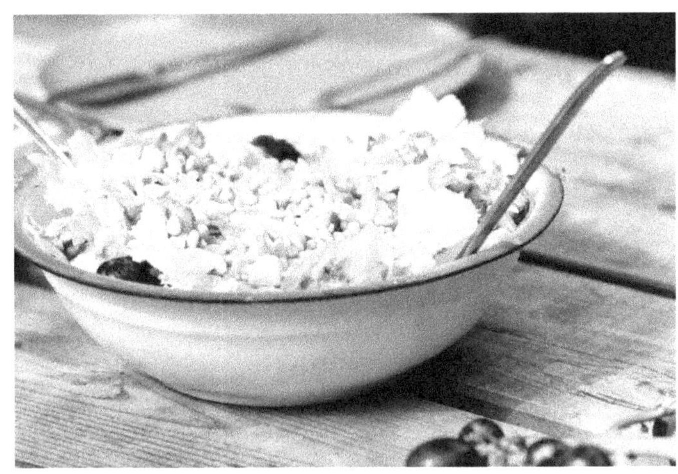

Yields Provided: 4 servings

Prep & Cook Time: 45-50 minutes

Nutritional Value Per Serving:

•	**Calorie Counts**	•	177
•	**Net Carbohydrates**	•	1 gram
•	**Protein**	•	2 grams
•	**Total Fats**	•	7 grams

Ingredients - The Salad:

- Small cauliflower (1 - divided)
- Small Romanesco cauliflower (1 - divided)
- Broccoli (1 lb.)
- Seedless oranges (2)

Ingredients - The Vinaigrette:

- Finely chopped anchovies (4)
- Orange juice & zest (1)
- Salted – unrinsed capers (1 tbsp.)
- Finely chopped hot pepper (1)
- Pepper & Salt (to your liking)
- Extra-virgin olive oil (4 tbsp.)

Prep Technique:

1. Cut the cauliflower into florets. Remove the peel and thinly slice the oranges. Finely chop the anchovies, capers, and hot peppers for the vinaigrette.
2. Prepare the vinaigrette fixings in a jar with a lid. Shake well and set aside.
3. Set up the Instant Pot with one cup of water and the steamer basket. Add the cauliflower to the basket and secure the lid. Set the timer for 6

minutes using low pressure. Quick-release the steam pressure when you hear the buzzer.

4. Toss the florets into a serving bowl with the prepared oranges. Toss.

5. Drizzle with the vinaigrette and serve.

Greek Salad

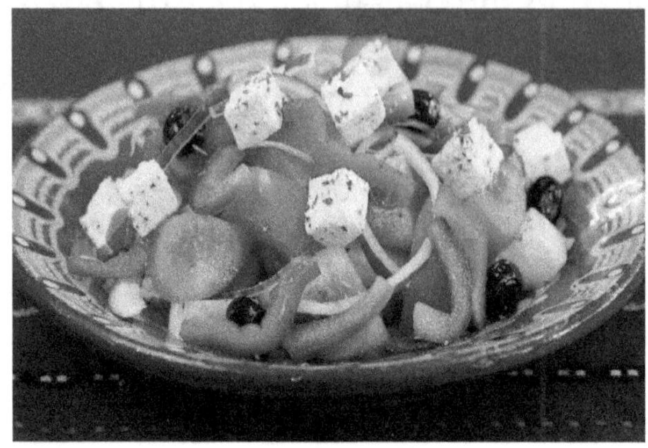

Yields Provided: 1 serving

Prep & Cook Time: 10-15 minutes

Nutritional Value Per Serving:

• **Calorie Counts**	•	594
• **Net Carbohydrates**	•	8 grams
• **Protein**	•	12 grams
• **Total Fats**	•	58 grams

Ingredients:

- Tomato (.25 cup)
- Bell pepper (.25 cup)
- Olives (1 tbsp.)
- Red onion (.25 cup)
- Cucumber (.25 cup)
- Olive oil (3 tbsp.)
- Feta cheese (.5 cup)
- Red wine vinegar (.5 tbsp.)
- Black pepper and salt (as desired)

Prep Technique:

1. Dice the tomato, chop the olives, and slice the onion, cucumber, and pepper. Combine the bell pepper, tomato, cucumber, crumbled feta cheese, and onion.
2. Spritz using the oil and vinegar with a shake of pepper and salt to your liking.
3. Toss until all of the fixings are well mixed before serving.

Soup Choices

Broccoli Curry Soup

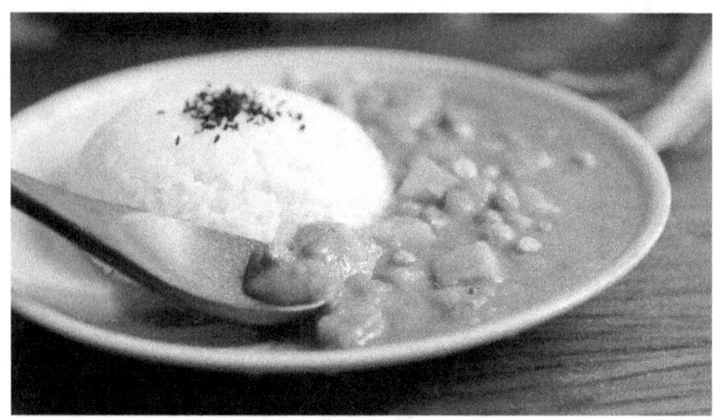

Yields Provided: 4 servings

Prep & Cook Time: 30-35 minutes

Nutritional Value Per Serving:

•	**Calorie Counts**	•	375
•	**Net Carbohydrates**	•	5 grams
•	**Protein**	•	17 grams
•	**Total Fats**	•	20 grams

Ingredients:

- Salt & Black pepper (as needed)
- Onion (1 chopped)
- Curry (1 tbsp.)
- Coconut oil (2 tbsp.)
- Vegetable stock (1 liter)
- Coconut cream (1 cup)
- Cheese substitute - your choice (75 g grated)
- Broccoli (1 lb.)

Prep Technique:

1. Pour coconut oil into a frying pan on the stovetop using the med-high heat setting.
2. Mix in the onion. Simmer for approximately six minutes.
3. Lower the temperature to medium. Then, add in the broth until it begins to simmer. Mix in the broccoli as well as any seasonings before adding curry. Simmer for 20 minutes.
4. Pour into a blender before mixing in the cheese substitute.
5. Blend well.

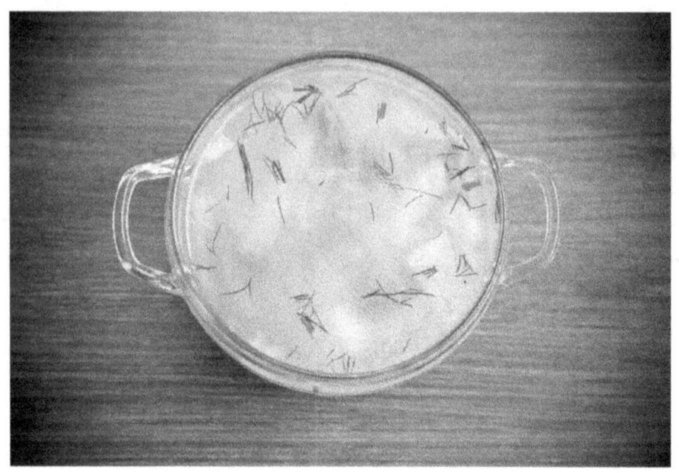

Yields Provided: 4 servings

Prep & Cook Time: 4-9 hours – varies

Nutritional Value Per Serving:

•	**Calorie Counts**	•	457
•	**Net Carbohydrates**	•	7.5 grams
•	**Protein**	•	40 grams
•	**Total Fats**	•	29 grams

Ingredients:

- Garlic clove (1)
- Cilantro (1 tbsp.)
- Small onion (1)
- Cream cheese (8 oz.)
- Chicken broth (1 cup)
- Chicken breasts – skinless & boneless (1 lb.)
- Diced tomatoes (14 oz.)
- Diced jalapeno (.5 oz.)
- Freshly squeezed lime juice (1.6 oz)
- Black pepper (1 tbsp.)
- Salt (1 tsp.)

Prep Technique:

1. Chop the garlic and cilantro. Dice the onion and jalapeno.
2. Combine all of the fixings in the crockpot. Prepare on the low-temperature setting for 6-9 hours or high for four hours.
3. Once it is done, shred the chicken in the pot using two forks.
4. Serve.

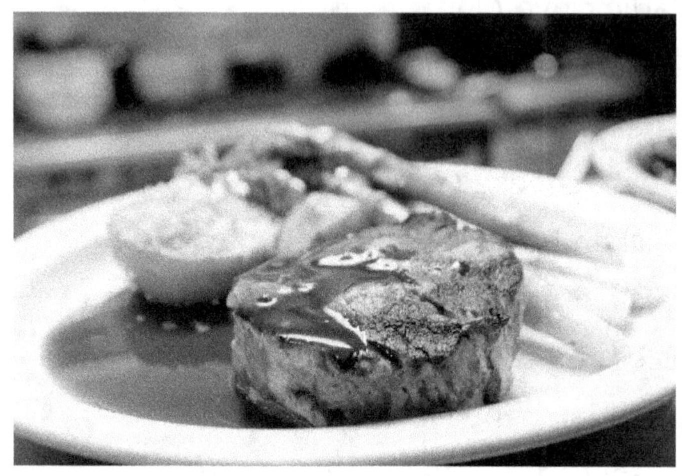

Yields Provided: 8 servings

Prep & Cook Time: 30 minutes

Nutritional Value Per Serving:

• **Calorie Counts**	• 326
• **Net Carbohydrates**	• 8 grams
• **Protein**	• 23 grams
• **Total Fats**	• 17 grams

Ingredients:

- Chopped onion – 1 medium or Dried onion flakes (.5 cup)
- Beef (2 lbs.)
- Tomato sauce (2 – 15 oz. cans)
- Tabasco sauce (1 tsp.)
- Tomato paste (6 oz.)
- Garlic powder (1 tsp.) or Minced cloves (2)
- Chili powder (.5 tbsp.)
- Cumin powder (2 tbsp.)
- Dried oregano (1 tsp.)
- Fine ground sea salt (2 tsp.)
- Chicken or beef broth (as needed for thinning)

Prep Technique:

1. Finely chop the onion. Use the sauté function on the Instant Pot to brown the hamburger. Blend in the Tabasco, onion flakes, cumin, salt, chili powder, and oregano. Mix thoroughly. Empty one cup of the broth over the burger, but do *not* stir.
2. Pour in the tomato sauce and paste - but do *not* stir.
3. Close the top and use the manual high-pressure setting for 10 minutes. When done, merely

natural-release the built-up pressure for 10 minutes, then quick-release.

4. Stir and serve.

Dinner Menu Options

Avocado & Salmon Omelet Wrap

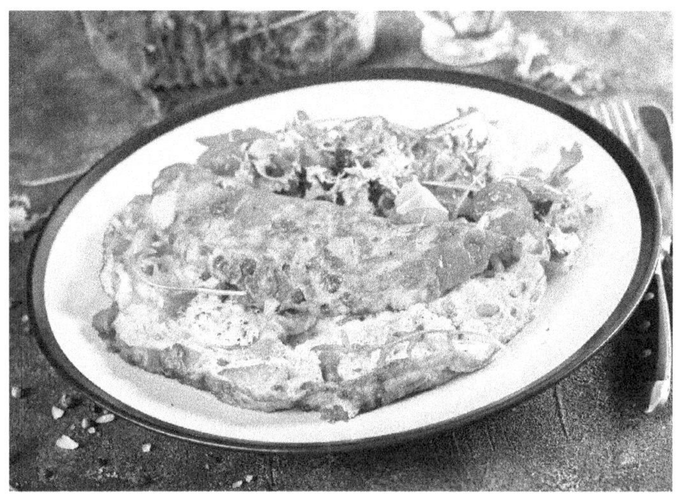

Yields Provided: 2 servings

Prep & Cook Time: 10-15 minutes

Nutritional Value Per Serving:

•	**Calorie Counts**	•	765
•	**Net Carbohydrates**	•	6 grams
•	**Protein**	•	37 grams
•	**Total Fats**	•	67 grams

Ingredients:

- Large eggs (3)
- Smoked salmon (1.8 oz.)
- Avocado (.5 of 1 average-size)
- Spring onion (1)
- Cream cheese - full-fat (2 tbsp)
- Chives - freshly chopped (2 tbsp.)
- Butter or ghee (1 tbsp.)
- Pepper and salt (as desired)

Prep Technique:

1. Add a sprinkle of pepper and salt to the eggs. Use a fork or whisk—mixing them well. Blend in the chives and cream cheese.
2. Prepare the salmon and avocado (peel and slice or chop).
3. Combine the butter/ghee and the egg mixture in a frying pan. Continue cooking on low heat until done.
4. Place the omelet on a serving dish with a portion of cheese over it. Sprinkle the onion, prepared avocado, and salmon into the wrap.
5. Close and serve!

BBQ Chicken Zucchini Boats

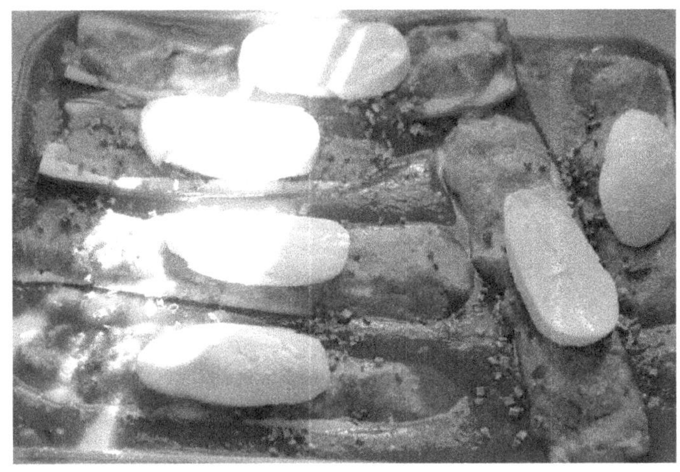

Yields Provided: 4 servings

Prep & Cook Time: 40 minutes

Nutritional Value Per Serving:

• **Calorie Counts**	• 212
• **Net Carbohydrates**	• 9 grams
• **Protein**	• 19 grams
• **Total Fats**	• 11 grams

Ingredients:

- Zucchini (3 halved)
- Chicken breast (1 lb. cooked)
- BBQ sauce (.5 cup)
- Shredded Mexican cheese (.33 cup)
- Avocado (1 sliced)
- Halved cherry tomatoes (.5 cup)
- Diced green onions (.25 cup)
- Keto-friendly ranch dressing (3 tbsp.)
- Also Needed: 9x13 casserole dish

Prep Technique:

1. Set the oven to reach 350° Fahrenheit.
2. Use a sharp knife and cut the zucchini in half. Discard the seeds. Make the boat by carving out of the center. Place the zucchini flesh side up into the casserole dish.
3. Discard and cut the skin and bones from the chicken. Shred and add the chicken in with the barbeque sauce. Toss to coat all the chicken.
4. Fill the zucchini boats with the mixture using about .25 to .33 cup each.
5. Sprinkle with Mexican cheese on top.

6. Bake for approximately 15 minutes. (If you would like it tenderer; bake for an additional 5 to 10 minutes to reach the desired tenderness.)

7. Remove from the oven. Top it off with avocado, green onion, tomatoes, and a drizzle of dressing. Serve.

Beetroot-Cured Salmon With Dill Oil

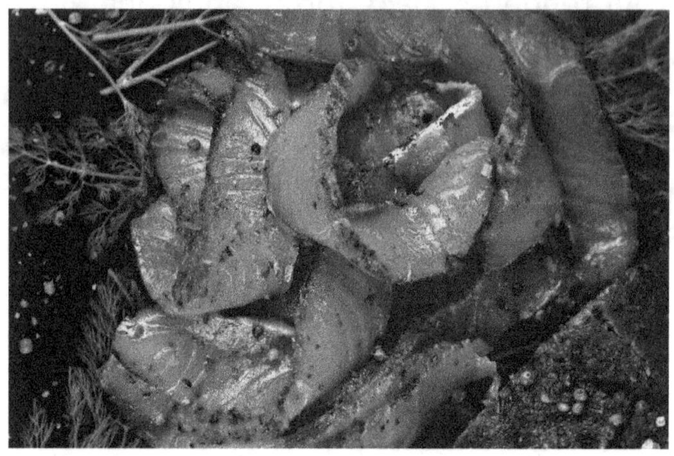

Yields Provided: 4 servings

Prep & Cook Time: 1-2 days – varies

Nutritional Value Per Serving:

•	**Calorie Counts**	•	500
•	**Net Carbohydrates**	•	4 grams
•	**Protein**	•	25 grams
•	**Total Fats**	•	42 grams

Ingredients:

- Beet (1)
- Salt (2 tbsp.)
- White peppercorns (5)
- Lime - zested (1)
- Salmon (1 lb.)

Ingredients - Dill Oil:

- Chopped fresh dill (.5 cup)
- Frozen spinach (1 tbsp.)
- Light olive oil or avocado oil (.5 cup)
- Salt and pepper (to your liking)

Ingredients - Serving:

- Daikon - finely sliced (2 oz.)
- Lettuce (.5 lb.)

Prep Technique:

1. Rinse the beetroot thoroughly and peel. Grate it coarsely and add it to a bowl along with the salt, peppercorn, and lime zest.
2. Partially defrost the salmon before the curing process.
3. Arrange the salmon with the skin side down and rub the flesh side evenly through the beetroot mixture. (You should probably wear a pair of

gloves on your hands to prevent staining.)

4. Arrange the salmon in a glass dish with a piece of film over the top. Marinate in the fridge for one to two days, flipping halfway through the process.

5. Combine the spinach and dill with a hand blender. Mix in the oil, salt, and pepper.

6. Unwrap the salmon and brush off the beetroot cure (don't serve the marinade).

7. Cut the fish into thin slices and serve with a portion of dill oil, chopped bacon, and leafy greens.

Cheeseburger Calzone

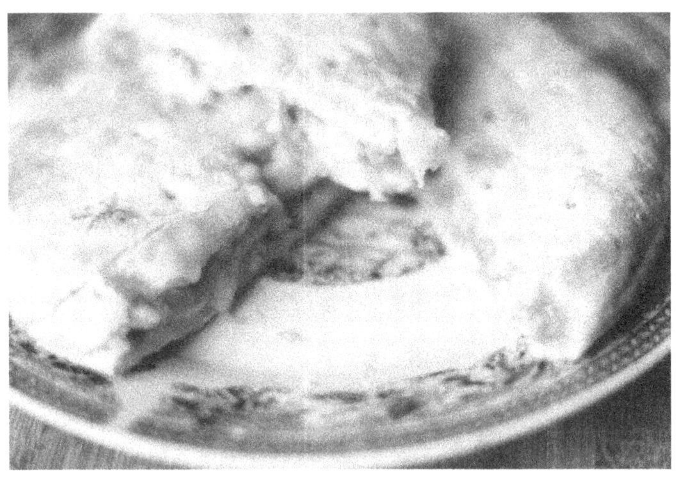

Yields Provided: 8 servings

Prep & Cook Time: 45-50 minutes

Nutritional Value Per Serving:

•	**Calorie Counts**	•	580
•	**Net Carbohydrates**	•	3 grams
•	**Protein**	•	34 grams
•	**Total Fats**	•	47 grams

Ingredients:

- Dill pickle spears (4)
- Cream cheese – divided (8 oz.)
- Shredded mozzarella cheese (1 cup)
- Egg (1)
- Yellow diced onion (.5 of 1)
- Ground beef - lean (1.5 lb.)
- Thick-cut bacon strips (4)
- Almond flour (1 cup)
- Mayonnaise (.5 cup)
- Shredded cheddar cheese (1 cup)

Prep Technique:

1. Program the oven temperature setting to 425º Fahrenheit. Prepare a cookie tin with parchment paper.
2. Chop the pickles into spears. Set aside for now.
3. Prepare the crust. Combine half of the cream cheese and mozzarella cheese. Microwave it for 35 seconds. When it melts, add the egg and almond flour to make the dough. Set aside.
4. Cook the beef on the stovetop using the medium heat setting.

5. Prepare the bacon until crunchy (microwave for five minutes or stovetop). When cool, break into bits.

6. Dice the onion and add to the beef. Cook until softened. Toss in the bacon, cheddar cheese, pickle bits, the rest of the cream cheese, and mayonnaise. Stir well.

7. Roll the dough onto the prepared baking tin. Scoop the mixture into the center. Fold the ends and side to make the calzone.

8. Bake it until browned or about 15 minutes. Let it rest for 10 minutes before slicing.

Fettuccine Chicken Alfredo

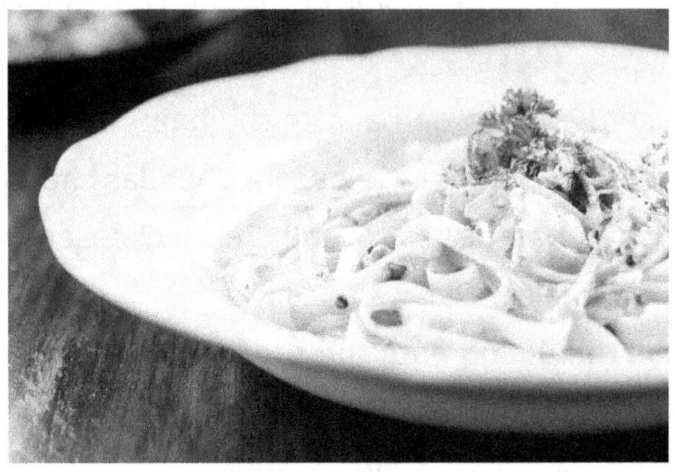

Yields Provided: 2 servings

Prep & Cook Time: 25-30 minutes

Nutritional Value Per Serving:

•	**Calorie Counts**	•	585
•	**Net Carbohydrates**	•	1 gram
•	**Protein**	•	25 grams
•	**Total Fats**	•	51 grams

Ingredients:

- Butter (2 tbsp.)
- Minced garlic cloves (2)
- Dried basil (.5 tsp.)
- Heavy cream (.5 cup)
- Grated parmesan (4 tbsp.)

Ingredients - The Chicken & Noodles

- Chicken thighs - no bones or skin (2)
- Olive oil (1 tbsp.)
- Miracle Noodle - Fettuccini (1 bag)
- Black pepper & salt (as desired)

Prep Technique:

1. *For the Sauce*: Measure and toss the butter and cloves into a pan. Sauté for two minutes. Pour the cream into the skillet and simmer two additional minutes.
2. Toss in one tablespoon of the parmesan at a time. Add the pepper, salt, and dried basil. Simmer 3 to 5 minutes on the low-heat temperature setting.
3. *For the Chicken*: Pound the chicken with a meat tenderizer hammer until it's ½-inch thick. Warm up the oil in a frying pan using the medium heat

setting. Toss in the chicken to simmer for approximately seven minutes per side. Shred and set aside.

4. *For the Noodles*: Prepare the package of noodles. Boil them for two minutes in a pot of water.

5. Fold in the noodles along with the sauce and shredded chicken. Cook slowly for two minutes and serve.

Fish Cakes

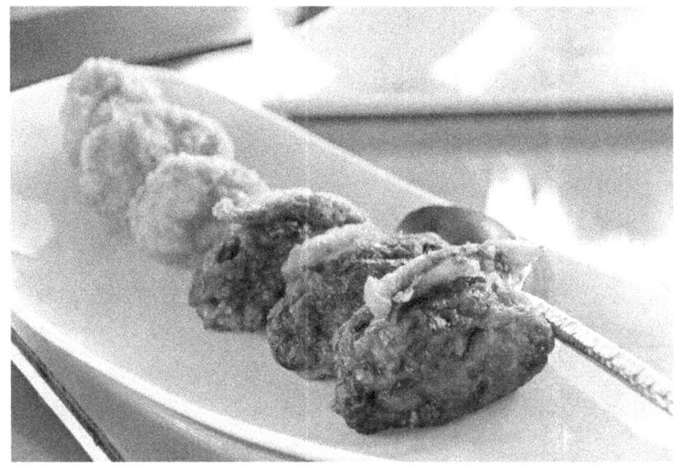

Yields Provided: 6 servings

Prep & Cook Time: 20-25 minutes

Nutritional Value Per Serving:

•	**Calorie Counts**	•	69
•	**Net Carbohydrates**	•	0.6 grams
•	**Protein**	•	1.1 grams
•	**Total Fats**	•	6.5 grams

Ingredients:

- Wild-caught raw white boneless fish (1 lb.)
- Cilantro - leaves and stems (.25 cup)
- Pinch of salt (1 pinch)
- Chili flakes (1 pinch)
- Coconut oil/ ghee - for frying (1-2 tbsp.)
- Avocado or a neutral oil - for greasing your hands (as needed)
- Avocados (2 ripe)
- Lemon (1 juiced)
- Salt (1 pinch)
- Water (2 tbsp.)
- Optional: Garlic cloves (1-2)
- Also Needed: Blender or food processor

Prep Technique:

1. Toss the fish, herbs, garlic, salt, chili, and fish into a food processor. Blitz until everything is combined evenly.
2. Using the med-high heat setting and add the ghee or coconut oil into a large skillet. Swirl the pan to coat.
3. Oil your hands and roll the fish mixture into six patties.

4. Add the cakes to the heated frying pan. Simmer until golden brown.

5. While the fish cakes are cooking, add all of the dipping sauce fixings (starting with the lemon juice) into a blender. Blitz until creamy. Taste the mixture and add more lemon juice or salt if desired.

6. When the fish cakes are cooked, serve warm with dipping sauce.

Ground Beef Veggie Skillet

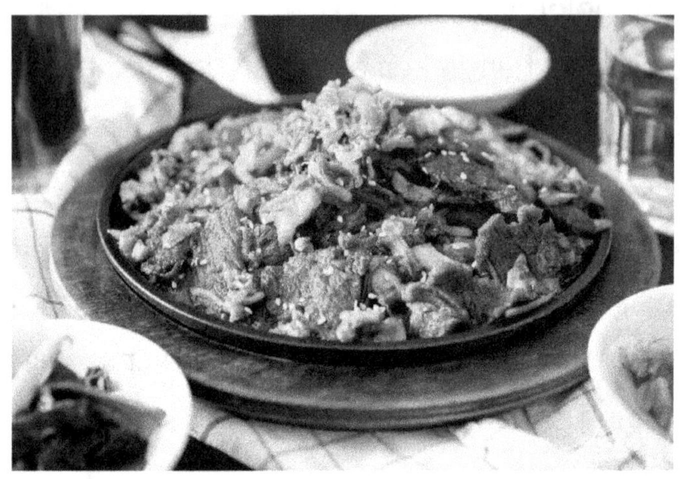

Yields Provided: 4 servings

Prep & Cook Time: 30-35 minutes

Nutritional Value Per Serving:

• **Calorie Counts**	•	261
• **Net Carbohydrates**	•	6 grams
• **Protein**	•	30 grams
• **Total Fats**	•	13 grams

Ingredients:

- Clove of garlic (1)
- Onions (.5 cup)
- Red bell peppers (.5 cup)
- Zucchini (1 medium)
- Asparagus (.5 lb.)
- Extra-virgin olive oil (2 tbsp.)
- Extra-lean ground beef (1 lb.)
- Dijon mustard (1 tsp.)
- Tomato passata or tomato sauce (.25 cup)
- Dried oregano (.5 tsp.)
- *Optional*: Crushed red pepper (.125 tsp.)
- Black pepper & salt (as desired)
- *Toppings*:
- Crumbled feta cheese (1 tbsp.)
- Freshly chopped parsley (as desired)

Prep Technique:

1. Mince or dice the garlic, onions, and peppers. Quarter the zucchini and slice the asparagus into three segments each.
2. Heat a large skillet using the med-high heat setting and pour in the olive oil.

3. Toss in the garlic and beef. Break apart as it is cooking. Stir occasionally and cook for about seven minutes until it's no longer pink. Transfer the meat from the skillet and set aside for now.

4. Fold in the onions and red bell peppers, and simmer until the onions are softened or about three to four minutes. Pour in a little bit of olive oil to sauté the veggies - as needed.

5. Toss in the zucchini and asparagus. Simmer for another three to five minutes.

6. Return the beef to the skillet and mix everything well.

7. Simmer for one to two additional minutes.

8. Garnish with fresh parsley and feta cheese.

Tasty Fat Bombs

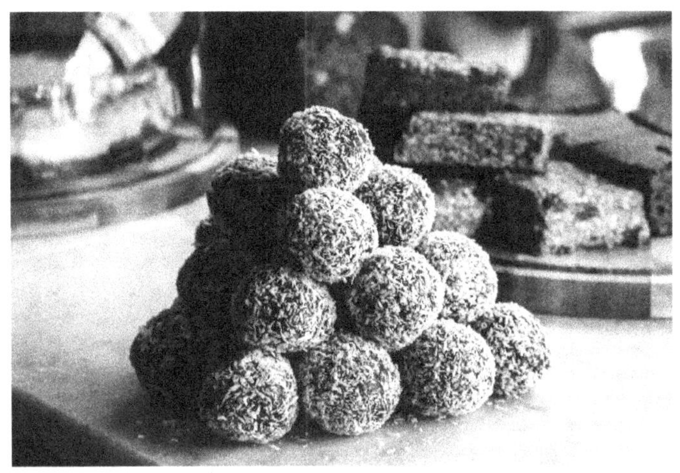

Blueberry Frozen Fat Bombs

Yields Provided: 24 servings

Prep & Cook Time: 10 minutes + freeze time

Nutritional Value Per Serving:

•	**Calorie Counts**	•	116
•	**Net Carbohydrates**	•	1.02 grams
•	**Protein**	•	.44 grams
•	**Total Fats**	•	13 grams

Ingredients:

- Scant blueberries (1 cup)
- Butter (1 stick)
- Coconut oil (.75 cup)
- Softened cream cheese (4 oz.)
- Coconut cream (.25 cup)
- Sweetener of choice (to taste)

Prep Technique:

1. Arrange three to four berries in each mold cup.
2. Melt the butter with the coconut oil over the lowest stovetop heat setting. Cool slightly for approximately five minutes.
3. Combine all of the ingredients and whisk well. Slowly, add the sweetener.
4. Using a spouted pitcher, fill an ice tray with 24 bombs.
5. Pop them out and eat when hunger strikes.

Cheesy Bacon Bombs

Yields Provided: 20 servings

Prep & Cook Time: 15-20 minutes

Nutritional Value Per Serving:

•	**Calorie Counts**	•	89
•	**Net Carbohydrates**	•	0.6 grams
•	**Protein**	•	5 grams
•	**Total Fats**	•	7.2 grams

Ingredients:

- Bacon (10 slices)
- Mozzarella cheese (8 oz.)
- Melted butter (4 tbsp.)
- Almond flour (4 tbsp.)
- Psyllium husk powder (3 tbsp.)
- Large egg (1)
- Sea salt (.25 tsp.)
- Onion powder (.125 tsp.)

- Garlic powder (.125 tsp.)
- Black pepper (.25 tsp.)
- Lard or oil for frying (1 cup)

Prep Technique:

1. Warm up the oil/lard until it reaches 350º Fahrenheit in a pan or fryer.
2. Add about half the cheese into a microwavable dish and cook for 45 to 60 seconds until melted.
3. For the butter, microwave 15 to 20 seconds, and add to the cheese along with the egg.
4. Blend in the almond flour, psyllium husk, and spices. Arrange the dough on a silicone mat and roll out into a rectangular shape.
5. Add the remainder of cheese and fold to form a rectangle. Slice into 20 squares.
6. Wrap each segment with 1/2 slices of bacon and secure with a toothpick.
7. Cook each of the fat bombs (3-4 at a time) until crispy.
8. Remove the bombs from the oil, drain, and serve.

Stuffed Pecan Fat Bombs

Yields Provided: 1 serving

Prep & Cook Time: 20 minutes

Nutritional Value Per Serving:

•	**Calorie Counts**	•	150
•	**Net Carbohydrates**	•	2 grams
•	**Protein**	•	11 grams
•	**Total Fats**	•	31 grams

Ingredients:

- Pecan halves (4)
- Cream cheese (1 oz.)
- Coconut butter/unsalted butter (.5 tbsp.)
- Sea salt (1 pinch)
- Your favorite flavor mix – herb or veggie

Prep Technique:

1. Warm up the oven to 350º Fahrenheit. Once it's hot, toast the pecans for 8 to 10 minutes. Cool.

2. Let the cream cheese and butter soften. Add the mixture with your favorite flavored mix, veggie, or herbs. Mix until smooth.

3. Spread the tasty fixings between the two pecan halves.

4. Drizzle with some sea salt and serve.

Dessert Favorites

Avocado & Chocolate Pudding

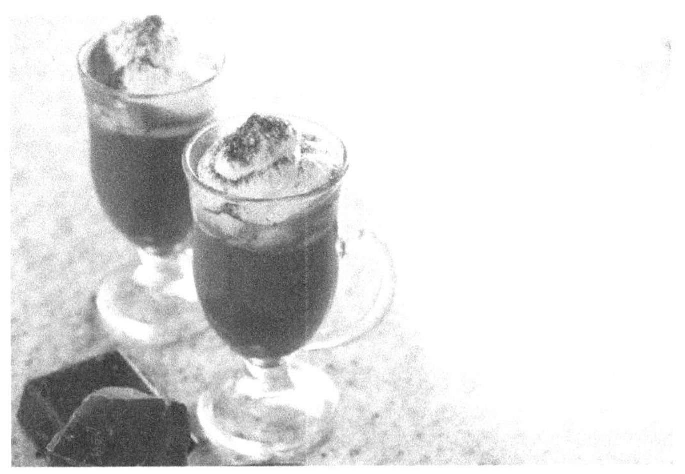

Yields Provided: 2 servings

Prep & Cook Time: 30 minutes

Nutritional Value Per Serving:

•	**Calorie Counts**	•	281
•	**Net Carbohydrates**	•	2 grams
•	**Protein**	•	8 grams
•	**Total Fats**	•	27 grams

Ingredients:

- Unchilled cream cheese (2 oz.)
- Ripe medium avocado (1)
- Natural sweetener – swerve (1 tsp.)
- Vanilla extract (.25 tsp.)
- Unsweetened cocoa powder (4 tbsp.)
- Pink salt (1 pinch)

Prep Technique:

1. Combine the cream cheese with the avocado, sweetener, vanilla, cocoa powder, and salt into the blender or processor.
2. Pulse until creamy smooth.
3. Measure into a fancy dessert dishes and chill for at least 30 minutes.

Banana Split Cheesecake

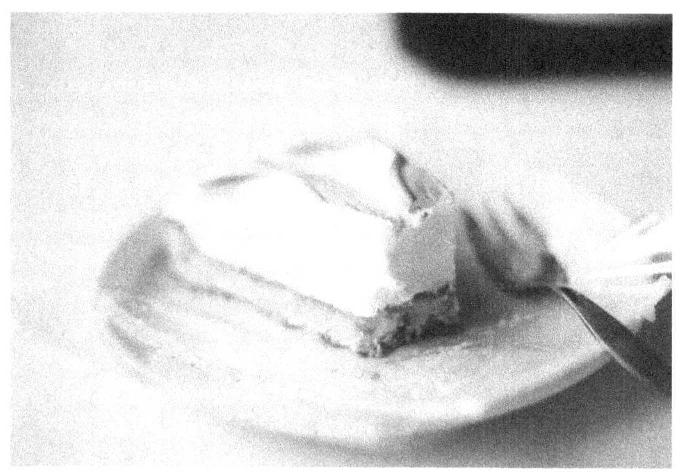

Yields Provided: 20 servings

Prep & Cook Time: 15-20 minutes

Nutritional Value Per Serving:

•	**Calorie Counts**	•	302
•	**Net Carbohydrates**	•	7 grams
•	**Protein**	•	4 grams
•	**Total Fats**	•	30 grams

Ingredients - The Crust:

- Cinnamon (2 tsp.)
- Almond flour (3 cups)
- Swerve (.33 cup)
- Melted butter (1 cup)
- *Also Needed*: 9 x 13-inch pan

Ingredients - The Filling:

- Swerve confectioner's sugar (1 cup)
- Melted butter (1 cup)
- Cream cheese (16 oz.)

Ingredients - The Topping:

- Chopped banana (1)
- Sliced strawberries (2 pints)
- Lemon juice (1 tbsp.)
- Heavy whipping cream (2 cups)
- Gelatin (1.5 tsp.)
- Vanilla extract (1 tsp.)
- Swerve (3 tbsp.)
- Water (3 tbsp.)
- *Optional:* Chocolate sauce & Nuts

Prep Technique:

1. Combine the crust fixings and press together in the pan.
2. Melt the butter and mix with the sweetener and cream cheese until creamy. Spread on top of the crust.
3. Combine the strawberries and banana in a mixing dish along with the lemon juice. Make the next layer.
4. Prepare the topping. Combine the whipping cream and gelatin in the water and beat well. Blend in the vanilla extract and sweetener. Whip until it is creamy to cover and make the next layer.
5. Top with the chocolate sauce and nuts if you like it that way.

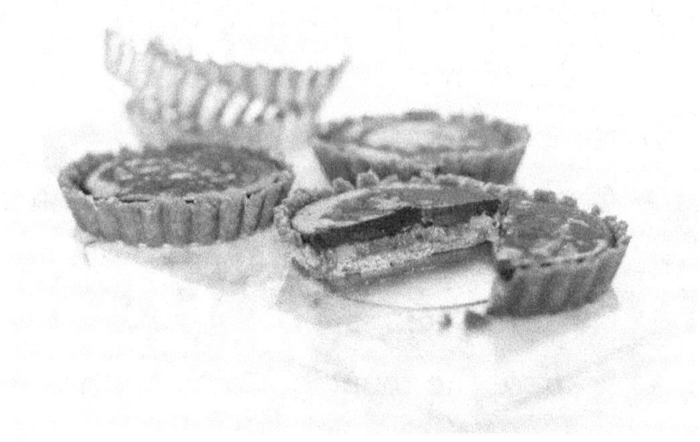

Yields Provided: 8 servings

Prep & Cook Time: 10 minutes + chill time

Nutritional Value Per Serving:

•	Calorie Counts	•	223
•	Net Carbohydrates	•	3 grams
•	Protein	•	6 grams
•	Total Fats	•	18 grams

Ingredients:

- Keto-friendly mini pie crusts (4)
- Melted coconut cream (2 tbsp.)
- Erythritol (as desired)
- Melted coconut oil (2 tbsp.)
- 100% chocolate - melted (2 oz.)
- Hazelnut butter (.25 cup)

Prep Technique:

1. Mix the coconut oil, coconut cream, chocolate, and erythritol in a mixing container.
2. Pour one tablespoon of the hazelnut butter in each tart crust.
3. Next, pour the chocolate mixture on top while filling up the tart crust.
4. Refrigerate for two hours until solid.

Pumpkin Bars With Cream Cheese Frosting

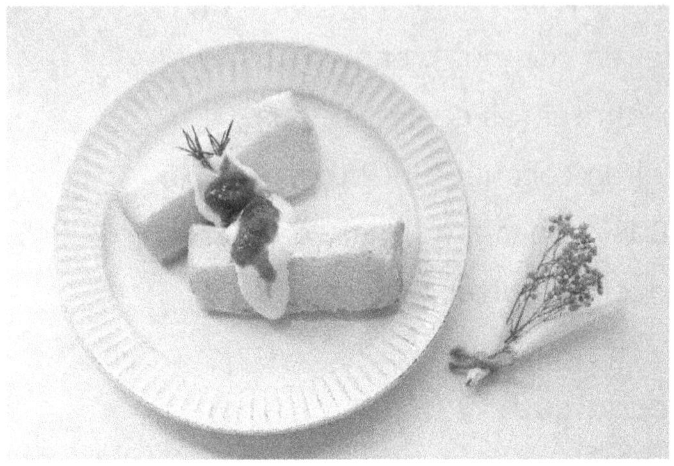

Yields Provided: 16 servings

Prep & Cook Time: 55-60 minutes

Nutritional Value Per Serving:

•	**Calorie Counts**	•	139
•	**Net Carbohydrates**	•	2 grams
•	**Protein**	•	3 grams
•	**Total Fats**	•	13 grams

Ingredients:

- Large eggs (2)
- Coconut oil (.25 cup)
- Cream cheese (2 oz.)
- Pumpkin puree (1 cup)
- Vanilla extract (1 tsp.)
- Erythritol sweetener blend (.66 cups
- Almond flour (1 cup)
- Pumpkin pie spice (1 tsp.)
- Sea salt (.5 tsp.)
- Gluten-free baking powder (2 tsp.)
- Also Needed: 9 x 9 baking pan

Ingredients - The Frosting:

- Powdered erythritol (.5 cup)
- Optional: Heavy cream (1 tbsp.)
- Softened cream cheese (6 oz.)
- Vanilla extract (1 tsp.)

Prep Technique:

1. Warm up the oven until it reaches 350º
   Fahrenheit. Cover the baking pan with
   parchment paper.

2. In a double boiler or microwave, melt the coconut oil and cream cheese.

3. Combine the vanilla, eggs, cream cheese mixture, and puree using a hand mixer until smooth using the medium-speed setting.

4. Whisk the dry fixings (salt, pie spice, baking powder, sweetener, and flour).

5. Mix all the ingredients with the mixer until just combined and pour into the pan.

6. Set the timer and bake for 20 to 30 minutes. Cool completely.

7. Prepare the frosting with each of the ingredients when the bars are cooled. If it's too thick, add a little cream or milk.

8. Slice into 16 equal portions. Enjoy any time.

Strawberry & Cream Cakes

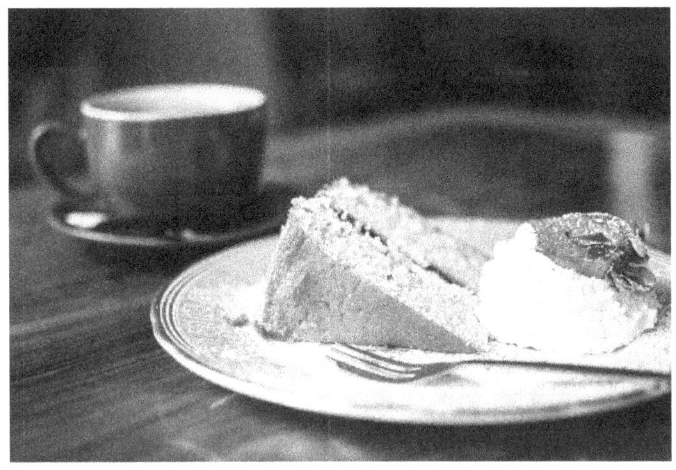

Yields Provided: 5 servings

Prep & Cook Time: 45 minutes

Nutritional Value Per Serving:

•	**Calorie Counts**	•	275
•	**Net Carbohydrates**	•	3.7 grams
•	**Protein**	•	6 grams
•	**Total Fats**	•	30 grams

Ingredients:

- Eggs (3)
- Cream cheese (3 oz./6 tbsp.)
- Vanilla extract (.5 tsp.)
- Baking powder (.25 tsp.)
- Erythritol (2 tbsp.)

Ingredients - The Filling:

- Strawberries (10)
- Heavy cream (1 cup)

Prep Technique:

1. Cover a baking sheet with parchment paper.
2. Break the eggs and which just the egg *whites.* Whisk to form stiff peaks.
3. In another dish, combine the cream cheese, egg *yolks*, vanilla extract, baking powder, and erythritol.
4. Slowly add the egg mixtures together and shape it into cake forms. Place them on the lined baking tin.
5. Whip the heavy cream until thickened.
6. Bake for 25-30 minutes.
7. Let them cool and add the berries and cream.

White Chocolate Bark

Yields Provided: 12 servings

Prep & Cook Time: 15-20 minutes

Nutritional Value Per Serving:

• **Calorie Counts**	• 40
• **Net Carbohydrates**	• 0 grams
• **Protein**	• 0 grams
• **Total Fats**	• 2 grams

Ingredients:

- Cocoa butter (.25 cup)
- Low-carb sweetener (.33 cup)
- Vanilla powder (1 tsp.)
- Hemp seed powder (.5 tsp.)
- Toasted pumpkin seeds (1 tsp.)
- Salt (as desired)
- Coconut oil - for the bowl

Prep Technique:

1. Chop the cocoa butter into little bits. Add water to a double boiler and add the pieces to melt using the medium heat setting. Stir in the rest of the fixings.
2. Lightly grease a bowl using a spritz of oil and add the mixture.
3. Let it cool and break into 12 portions.

Conclusion

Congratulations, you've reached the end of the book! You've learned quite a lot, and now it's time for you to start implementing everything you have learned and start seeing results!

Remember to pace yourself and increase your fasting periods in incremental steps, also use the recipes and my choice wholefoods listed in conjunction with exercise to achieve maximum results.

You've learned everything from the dark secrets of food manufactures designing habit-forming foods, intermittent fasting, mindful eating, chronic degenerative diseases, benefits of whole foods, exercise regiments, bio-hacks, body types, and even a little biochemistry.

You have everything you need to equip yourself on your weight loss journey. Remember, you are not alone in this journey and can reference this resource at any point in time if you're feeling stuck or need motivation.

I trust you are on your way to becoming the greatest version of yourself; you just need to follow through. I am wishing you a happy life full of abundance, longevity, peace of mind, health, and wellness.